Basic Techniques in Veterinary Parasitology and Molecular Biology

NIPA® GENX ELECTRONIC RESOURCES & SOLUTIONS P. LTD.
New Delhi-110 034

About the Authors

Angughali Aheto Sumi completed her master's in Food Biotechnology at the University of Abertay Dundee, Scotland, where she studied the role of circadian clock genes in potato tuberisation. She earned her PhD in Biomedicine from Universitat Pompeu Fabra, Barcelona, with her research based at the Centre for Genomic Regulation (CRG), focusing on biophysical mechanisms driving morphogenesis. After a bridging postdoc at CRG, she pursued further postdoctoral work at Institut Fresnel, Marseille, on the biophysics of large-scale cell migration. She is currently a research fellow at ICAR-NRC on Mithun, Jharnapani, Nagaland.

Dr. Jayanta Kumar Chamuah, born at Dhakuakhana, Lakhimpur district of a Assam, on 01-03-1979. He had completed BVSc & AH and MVSc in Veterinary Parasitology from College of Veterinary Science, Khanapara, Assam Agricultural University in 2002 and 2005; respectively. He was awarded University Merit Scholarship in both undergraduate and postgraduate degrees. He has completed PhD degree in Veterinary Parasitology from ICAR-Indian Veterinary Research Institute, Izatnagar-243122 in 2014. He was also awarded ICAR Net in 2008 and ARS in 2009 (Veterinary Parasitology) and also the recipient of ICAR-IVRI SRF for PhD in 2008. He has handled two External funded as a Principal Investigator and four as a Co-PI. He has also completed four institute projects as a Principal Investigated. He has published 20 international papers in a reputed Journal and 32 papers in National Journal. He prepared two technical bulletins, published two books and published four reviews in a reputed journal. He has registered two designs, seven copyrights registration to Intelectual Property Right office, Govt of India. Also three designs, three copyright, one trademark and one patents are under process in IPR office, Govt of India. He also commercialized two technologies to the stake holders. His interest in work is the molecular epidemiology of gastrointestinal parasites and proteomic works.

Dr. Binod Kumar obtained his B.V.Sc. and AH degrees from SVVU, Tirupati (College of Veterinary Science, Rajendranagar, Hyderabad) in 2008. He completed his postgraduate studies, both MVSc. and PhD, in Veterinary Parasitology from ICAR-Indian Veterinary Research Institute (IVRI), Izatnagar, Bareilly, in 2010 and 2016, respectively. He was awarded an IVRI Research Scholarship during MVSc and an ICAR Senior Research Fellowship during PhD. He served as Assistant Professor in the College of Veterinary Science and Animal Husbandry, Junagadh, Gujarat from 2012 to 2023, following he joined the College of Veterinary and Animal Science, Kishanganj, Bihar as Associate Professor in April 2023. He has published more than 60 research paper in peer-reviewed international journals and attended National and International seminars and symposia. He is also authored for five books and many book chapters. He is having a good knowledge of molecular parasitology and worked continuously for last 15 years on ticks and tick-borne diseases management in animals. He has successfully guided one MVSc and one Ph.D. student. He is awarded by 'Dr J. P. Dubey young scientist awards 2010' by IAAVP at Mumbai conference and Dr. N. S. Ruprah Memorial Oration Award-2023 by IAAVP at Hyderabad conference. Besides being reviewer to many scientific Journals, Dr. Binod Kumar is the Executive Council Member of Indian Association for Advancement of Veterinary Parasitology. Now-a-days he is actively engaged in teaching and institutional building activities at College of Veterinary and Animal Science, Kishanganj, Bihar.

Girish Patil S. completed MVSc and PhD from Indian Veterinary Research Institute (IVRI), Deemed University, Izatnagar. He further obtained MBA from Sikkim Manipal University of Distance Education and PGDTMA from University of Hyderabad and NAARM, Hyderabad. After working as Assistant Professor for 2 years, he joined National Academy of Agricultural Research Management, Hyderabad as Scientist, subsequently he was promoted to Senior Scientist (ICAR – National Research Centre on Pig, Rani, Guwahati) and Principal Scientist (ICAR - National Research Centre on Meat, Hyderabad). He currently holds the position of Director at ICAR NRC on Mithun, Jharnapani Nagaland.

Basic Techniques in Veterinary Parasitology and Molecular Biology

Volume 09: The Protocol Series

Angughali Aheto Sumi
Jayanta Kumar Chamuah
Binod Kumar
Girish Patil S.

NIPA® GENX ELECTRONIC RESOURCES & SOLUTIONS P. LTD.
New Delhi-110 034

NIPA® GENX ELECTRONIC RESOURCES & SOLUTIONS P. LTD.

101,103, Vikas Surya Plaza, CU Block
L.S.C. Market, Pitam Pura, New Delhi-110 034
Ph : +91-11-43860225, Mob.: +91 9717133558, 9540816132
E-mail: newindiapublishingagency@gmail.com
Website: www.nipaersources.com

Print ISBN: 978-93-58874-13-6
ebook ISBN: 978-93-58871-94-4

Composed and Designed by NIPA®.

Preface

This book has been prepared as a comprehensive guide for students and early-career researchers engaged in the study and diagnosis of animal parasitic diseases. The field of veterinary parasitology requires a solid foundation in both fundamental laboratory practices and specialised diagnostic techniques, and this manual aims to bridge that gap by providing clear, practical instructions for a wide range of essential procedures.

The manual opens with an overview of laboratory fundamentals and safety practices, including protocols for biosafety, proper equipment handling, waste management, and emergency response. Building on this foundation, it covers the preparation of laboratory solutions and reagents, equipping users with the necessary skills for routine and specialised work.

Subsequent chapters present step-by-step methods for diagnostic procedures in veterinary parasitology, including specimen collection, blood and faecal examinations, staining techniques, and microscopic analysis.

Recognising the growing importance of molecular biology in veterinary diagnostics, the manual also details standard protocols for DNA extraction, primer design, polymerase chain reaction (PCR), and sequence analysis. These advanced methods are becoming indispensable tools for the precise characterisation and identification of parasitic species.

To further support effective laboratory work, appendices provide practical checklists, troubleshooting guides, and recommendations for further reading and resources.

Whether you are a veterinary student beginning your laboratory journey or an early-career researcher, this manual is intended to serve as a valuable resource for basic lab skills. We hope that it will enhance both the quality and efficiency of laboratory investigations, ultimately contributing to improved animal health and disease management.

Authors

Acknowledgement

We would like to extend our heartfelt gratitude to the Director, ICAR-NRC on Mithun, Nagaland, for logistical support.

Authors

Contents

List of Tables

List of Figures

Introduction

This book provides an overview on laboratory fundamentals and basic techniques in veterinary parasitology and molecular biology. It is structured to provide a clear and practical understanding of essential methodologies, emphasising their principles and applications. The content is tailored for students and early career veterinary researchers with a foundational grasp of scientific concepts, ensuring accessibility without oversimplifying critical details.

Book Structure

Chapter 1: Laboratory Fundamentals and Safety Practices - This chapter focuses on the foundational aspects of laboratory work, ensuring safe and efficient practices. Topics include:

1. **General Lab Conduct**: Best practices for maintaining a professional and orderly laboratory environment. It includes equipment and instrument safety, waste management as well as emergency procedures.
2. **General Lab Equipment**: Overview of essential tools and their proper use.
3. **Preparation of Solutions and Reagents for Laboratory Use**

Chapter 2: Veterinary Parasitology Techniques- This chapter looks at essential techniques for studying and diagnosing parasitic infections in veterinary contexts. Topics covered include:

1. **Sample Collection and Preservation**: Best practices for collecting, transporting, and storing samples for parasitological studies.
2. **Routine blood examination**
3. **Staining and Microscopy Techniques**: Methods for visualising parasitic organisms under a microscope.
4. **Parasitological Examination Methods**: Techniques for identifying and quantifying parasitic organisms in biological samples.
5. **Serum Biochemistry and Immunodiagnostic Assays**

Chapter 3: Essential Techniques in Molecular Biology and Bioinformatics- This chapter introduces key techniques pivotal to modern molecular biology research and computational analysis. Topics include:

1. **Genomic DNA Extraction**: The foundational process of isolating DNA for various downstream applications.
2. **Primer Design with Primer3**: Guidelines and tools for designing primers essential for PCR-based experiments.
3. **Polymerase Chain Reaction (PCR) Amplification**: A cornerstone technique for amplifying DNA segments with precision.
4. **Sequence Alignment using MAFFT**: Methods for aligning genetic sequences to identify similarities and differences.

Appendix: To ensure laboratory efficiency, this manual includes an appendix covering:

- **Equipment Maintenance**: Guidelines for maintaining essential laboratory equipment.
- **Troubleshooting Guide**: Common challenges and solutions for the techniques outlined in this manual.

1

Laboratory Fundamentals and Safety Practices

This chapter introduces the essential components of laboratory work that form the foundation for veterinary parasitology and molecular biology research. A well-equipped laboratory along with proper safety protocols and correctly prepared reagents, is the key to reliable experimental outcomes and a secure working environment.

The following sections describe the standard operating procedures and laboratory biosafety, standard equipment used in research work, and the fundamental principles of solution preparation. These basic laboratory skills are essential prerequisites for the specialised techniques covered in subsequent chapters on veterinary parasitology, molecular biology and bioinformatics.

Understanding and applying these foundational concepts allows researchers to maintain experimental consistency, ensure reproducible results, and conduct investigations safely and efficiently. The methods and principles outlined here will be regularly applied throughout the various techniques detailed in this manual, serving as essential knowledge for all laboratory personnel as well short-term visitors.

1.1 Laboratory Standard Operating Procedures and Safety

Laboratory safety is fundamental to protecting personnel, maintaining sample integrity, and ensuring reliable experimental outcomes. This section outlines essential laboratory conduct, safety protocols for personnel and equipment, waste management, and emergency protocols for standard laboratories carrying out diagnostics as well as research.

1.1.1 General Laboratory Conduct and Biosafety Measures

Access control

Laboratory access is restricted to authorised staff only. This is because unauthorised persons may not be familiar with safety protocols and could disturb sensitive experiments. In molecular biology laboratories, this is particularly crucial as experiments requires strict contamination control. In parasitology labs, unauthorised persons might be exposed to potentially infectious materials.

Never eat, drink or apply cosmetics in the laboratory

This rule exists because laboratory surfaces and air may be contaminated with biological materials, chemicals, or aerosols that could be inadvertently ingested. Food and beverages can also become contaminated, creating serious health risks. Additionally, eating or drinking can interfere with molecular biology procedures by introducing nucleases from saliva or food particles that can degrade DNA/RNA samples.

Wear appropriate laboratory attire

Laboratory coats serve as the primary barrier between skin and hazardous materials. They should be worn at all times and removed before leaving the laboratory to prevent the spread of contaminants to common areas. Disposable gloves protect against biological materials, chemicals, and cross-contamination of samples. Different types of gloves may be required for specific procedures - latex or nitrile for general work, thick rubber gloves for handling concentrated chemicals, and thermal gloves for very hot or cold materials. Closed-toe shoes protect feet from chemical spills and dropped objects.

Personal hygiene and hand washing

Regular hand washing is crucial, particularly after handling specimens, before leaving the laboratory, and after removing gloves. Proper hand washing technique involves using warm water and soap for at least 20 seconds, paying attention to areas between fingers and under nails. This prevents the transfer of biological materials, including parasitic stages and microbial contaminants, that could affect personal health or PCR reactions.

Specimen container handling

Leaking or broken containers pose serious biosafety risks. They should never be opened as the contents may be hazardous and potentially aerosolised. Such incidents should be reported immediately to supervisors who can implement proper containment and decontamination procedures. This is particularly important when handling fecal samples for parasitology or blood/tissue samples for DNA extraction.

Culture and sample storage

Proper storage of cultures, specimens, and molecular biology reagents prevents accidents and maintains sample integrity. Tubes containing liquids should always be kept upright in appropriate racks to prevent spills. This is particularly important for molecular biology reagents and parasitological specimens that may contain infectious materials.

Chemical Handling

Proper chemical management includes maintaining updated Safety Data Sheets (SDS) and proper storage based on chemical compatibility. There should be regular inventory checks in order to keep track of chemicals that need to be replaced. Importantly, all solutions have to labelled properly and there should be appropriate disposal procedures in place.

Chemical or biological spills require immediate attention using appropriate cleanup protocols. For biological spills, sodium hypochlorite (10,000 ppm for high-risk materials, 1,000 ppm for general decontamination) is the primary disinfectant. The area should be covered with paper towels soaked in disinfectant, left for appropriate contact time, then cleaned while wearing proper PPE. All cleanup materials must be treated as biohazardous waste.

Data Security (Bioinformatics)

- Implement proper data backup procedures
- Maintain confidentiality of sensitive genetic data
- Use secure passwords and appropriate data encryption
- Regular updates of antivirus software
- Follow institutional guidelines for data storage and sharing

Health surveillance

Regular monitoring of laboratory personnel includes:

- Annual health checkups
- Vaccination of staff handling blood and blood products of zoonotic importance.
- Documentation of any work-related health issues
- Regular review of safety protocols

1.1.2 Equipment and Instrument Safety

Note: Please refer to Appendix A1 for more information on maintenance of key equipment

In order for laboratories to operate smoothly, it is mandatory to properly use and maintain crucial and sophisticated equipment. Whether it is a basic microscope or complex molecular analysis instrument, each piece of equipment requires specific handling protocols to ensure both user safety and experimental reliability. Proper equipment maintenance not only prevents accidents but also guarantees the accuracy of research results and longevity of laboratory instruments that are often expensive.

All users must undergo proper training before operating any laboratory equipment. This includes:

- Understanding of equipment-specific safety features and emergency shutoff procedures
- Knowledge of routine maintenance requirements
- Familiarity with troubleshooting common problems
- Understanding of equipment logs and proper documentation procedures
- Recognition of signs indicating equipment malfunction

1.1.3 Waste Management

The handling of laboratory waste in molecular biology and parasitology facilities requires careful attention to both safety and environmental considerations. Different types of waste present unique hazards and must be managed according to specific protocols to protect personnel, the environment, and comply with regulatory requirements.

1. Biohazardous Waste Management

- All materials contaminated with biological samples must be placed in designated red biohazard bags
- Double bagging required for wet waste to prevent leakage
- Bags must be properly labelled with date, laboratory origin, and type of waste
- Waste containers must have proper biohazard symbols and secure lids
- Regular autoclave validation using biological indicators
- Documentation of waste treatment and disposal

2. Chemical Waste Handling

- Segregation based on chemical compatibility
- Proper labelling with content and hazard information
- Use of appropriate containers resistant to stored chemicals
- Secondary containment for liquid waste
- Regular disposal through certified waste contractors
- Maintenance of disposal records and manifests

3. Molecular Biology Specific Waste

- Separate containers for materials containing ethidium bromide
- Special disposal protocols for acrylamide gels

- Proper handling of phenol chloroform waste
- Collection of restriction enzymes and other biological reagents
- Decontamination of nucleic acid-containing materials
- Specific protocols for radioactive material disposal if used

1.1.4 Emergency Procedures and Response Protocols

Laboratory emergencies require immediate and appropriate action to prevent injury and minimise damage. A comprehensive emergency preparedness plan is essential for maintaining safety in molecular biology and parasitology laboratories, where personnel may encounter various hazards including chemical exposures, biological contaminations, and equipment-related accidents.

Location and Maintenance of Emergency Equipment

Every laboratory member must be familiar with the location and proper use of emergency equipment:

- Emergency exits serve as primary evacuation routes and must remain unobstructed at all times, with clearly marked illuminated signs and updated evacuation maps posted throughout the facility. Regular testing of emergency lighting ensures functionality during power failures.
- Fire extinguishers are strategically placed throughout the laboratory, with different types available based on specific fire hazards. These undergo regular visual inspections for pressure and physical damage, with annual professional certification. Laboratory personnel should receive training in proper fire extinguisher usage techniques and fire response protocols.
- Eye wash stations and safety showers form critical emergency response infrastructure for chemical exposures. Eye wash stations must be located within 10 seconds' reach of areas where hazardous materials are handled. Safety showers, particularly important in areas handling corrosive chemicals must have adequate drainage systems.
- First aid kits contain supplies appropriate for laboratory-specific hazards. Regular inventory checks ensure supplies remain fully stocked and have not expired.
- Chemical spill kits contain appropriate absorbents and neutralisers for laboratory-specific chemicals, along with necessary personal protective equipment. Regular inventory checks should be carried out and updated according to requirement. Clear instructions for proper use should accompany each kit, enabling efficient response to chemical spills.

Emergency Communication Systems

Emergency contact information should be prominently displayed at laboratory entrances. This information includes contact numbers for the laboratory supervisor, biosafety officer (or similar person appointed by the institute), nearest emergency medical facility (such as hospitals), and facility maintenance. Regular updates ensure contact information remains current as personnel changes occur.

Incident Documentation and Response

All laboratory incidents, regardless of severity, require immediate documentation. Incident reports must detail the date, time, and location of the occurrence, personnel involved, description of the incident, actions taken, witnesses present, and any follow-up requirements. Regular review of incident reports helps identify patterns and implement preventive measures.

The laboratory should maintain detailed standard operating procedures for various emergency scenarios including chemical spills, biological material exposures, fire emergencies, medical emergencies, power failures, equipment malfunctions, and natural disasters. These procedures outline specific response protocols, chain of command, evacuation when necessary, documentation requirements, and follow-up actions.

Emergency Response Training

All laboratory personnel must complete emergency response training upon joining the laboratory and participate in refresher sessions. Such training should cover proper evacuation procedures, incident reporting protocols, and specific response procedures for various types of emergencies. Select personnel maintain first aid certification to ensure immediate response capability for medical emergencies.

1.2 General laboratory equipment

Laboratory equipment plays a vital role in the functioning of any diagnostic or research lab. These tools are essential for a wide range of tasks, including collecting, storing, transporting, and processing samples. In addition to handling samples, some equipment is specifically designed for the preparation and storage of lab supplies such as chemicals, reagents, plasticware, and glassware. Having the right tools ensures that lab work is conducted efficiently and accurately. The following section provides an overview of the ***essential and standard*** equipment required for setting up and operating a diagnostic or basic research lab.

<table>
<tr><td>Analytical Electronic Balance: For weighing of different chemicals for the preparation of media, reagents etc. Modern balances enable precise weighing, down to micrograms which is essential for sensitive experiments that require exact concentration of substrates. These balances often come with automation and calibration, which reduces human errors.</td><td>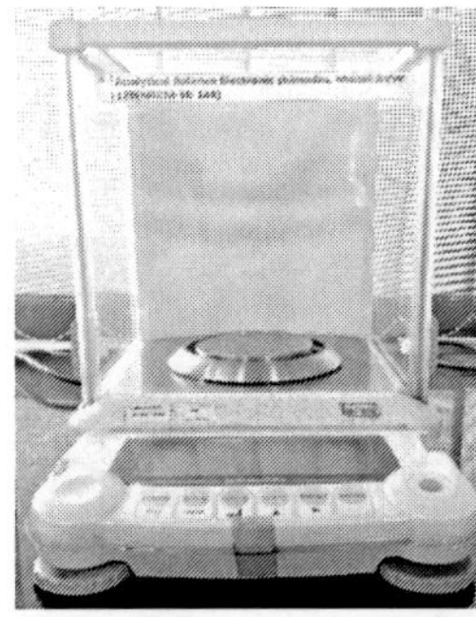
Fig. 1: Analytical electronic balance</td></tr>
<tr><td>Autoclave: A high-pressure steam equipment used to sterilise media, reagents, and other dry heat sensitive materials. Different kinds of medical/laboratory autoclaves are available in market based on size, automation, safety features, etc. Autoclaves are also used for biohazard waste decontamination.</td><td>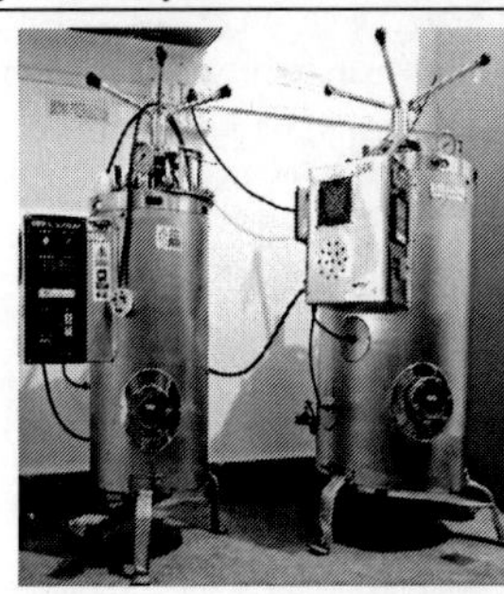
Fig. 2: Autoclaves (vertical)</td></tr>
<tr><td>Biosafety cabinet: An enclosed and ventilated workspace that protects both the laboratory personnel and surrounding environment from potentially harmful pathogens, it is mainly used for microbiological works.</td><td>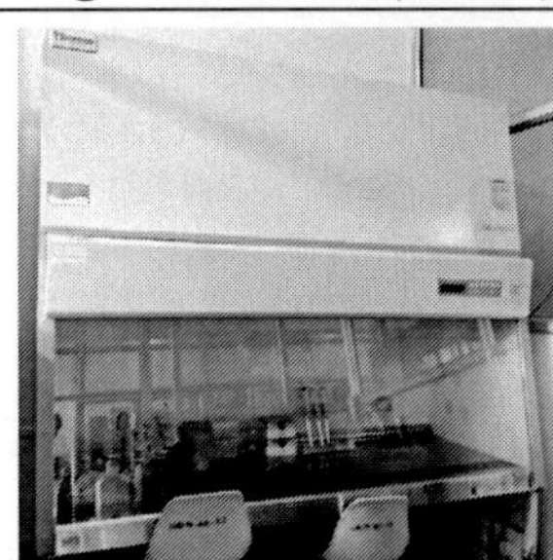
Fig. 3: Biosafety cabinet</td></tr>
<tr><td>Burner and Spirit Lamps: Used for flame-sterilising loops, needles, culture tubes and other items during bacterial culture work. At NRCM, sterile single-use plastic loops and spreaders are used inside a biosafety cabinet without the need for open flame sterilisation.</td><td>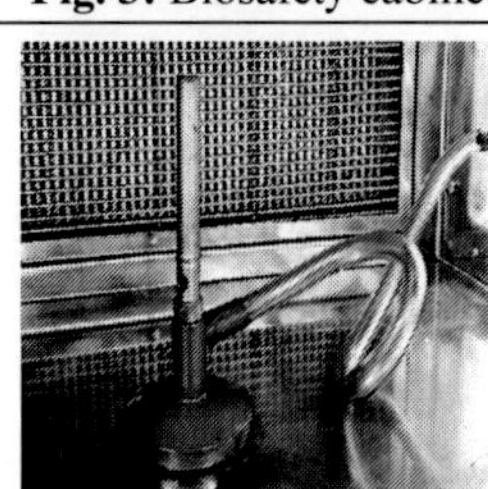
Fig. 4: Burner</td></tr>
</table>

Cold chain box: These are critical for transport of samples from field condition to the laboratory. These containers are used to preserve blood, tissue or microbial cultures as well as vaccines during transit to maintain their integrity and viability for further processing and use.	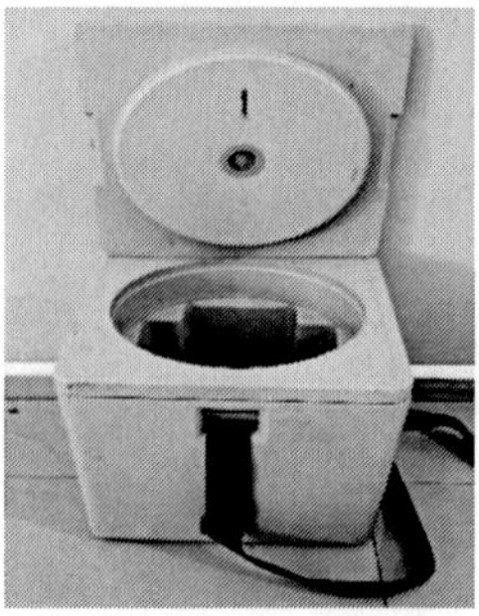 **Fig. 5:** Cold chain box
CO_2 Incubator: CO_2 incubators provide a controlled environment with specific CO_2 levels, humidity, and temperature, making them indispensable for culturing mammalian cells and anaerobic bacteria.	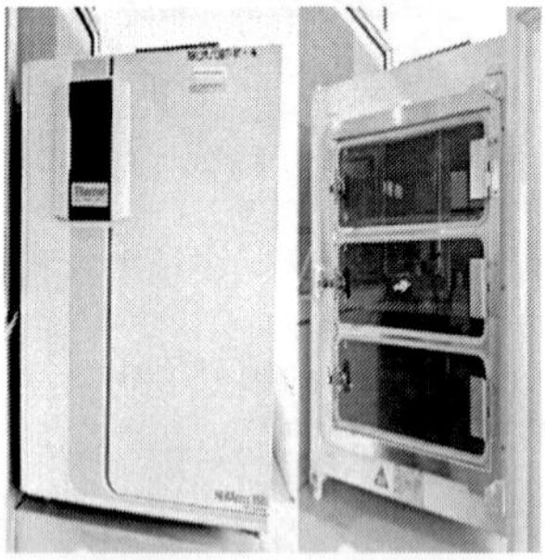 **Fig. 6:** CO_2 incubator
Deep Freezer: Deep freezers, usually operating at -20°C or -80°C, are crucial for long-term storage and preservation of biological samples, enzymes, and reagents. They prevent degradation of sensitive materials, such as RNA or vaccines. Deep freezers also help in maintaining viability of cell lines and microbial stocks used in research.	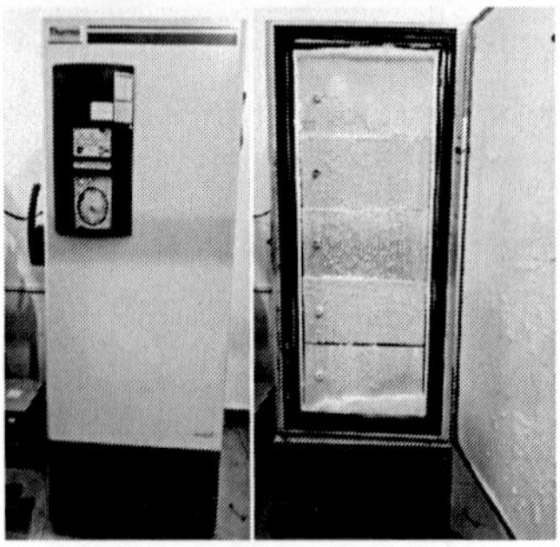 **Fig. 7:** Deep freezer (-80°C)
Desiccator: In veterinary research, a desiccator is essential for preserving tissue samples collected for histopathology by preventing moisture-induced degradation and for drying processed samples to ensure accurate analysis in diagnostic or experimental studies.	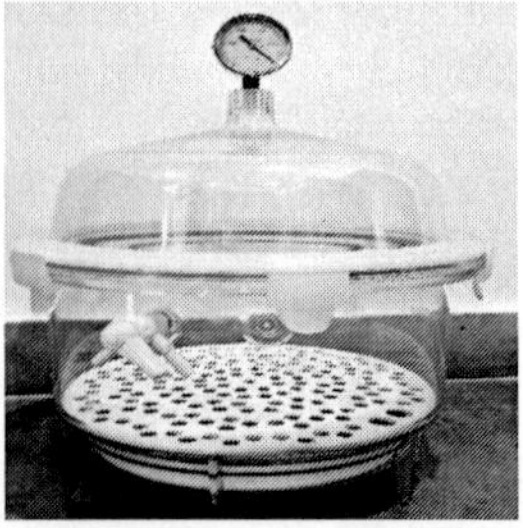 **Fig. 8:** Dessicator

Electrophoresis Unit: For carrying out separation of nucleic acid and protein based on size and charge for qualitative and quantitative analysis. These units are integral to molecular biology works such as visualisation of restriction enzyme digests, confirming PCR amplification, or analysing protein expression levels during SDS-PAGE work.	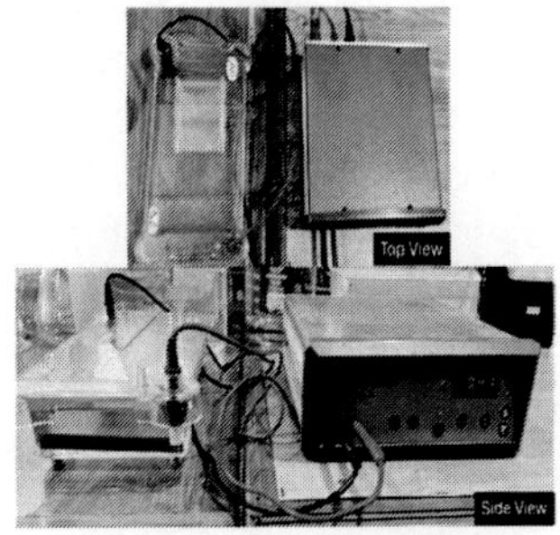 **Fig. 9:** Electrophoresis unit
ELISA Reader: ELISA readers **(Fig A)** allow for detection of antigens and antibodies in samples with high sensitivity and accuracy and are hence indispensable in serological work. Modern readers come with additional features such as automated plate washer (**Fig B**), built-in stabiliser and shaker that provide variable speeds and duration as per experiment requirements.	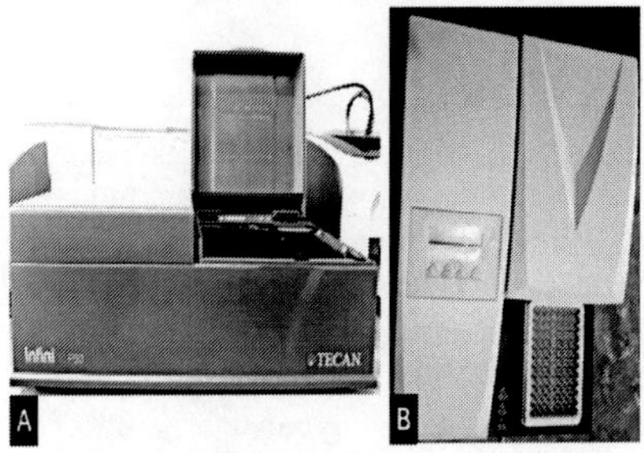 **Fig. 10:** ELISA reader
Gel Documentation System: For visualisation and documentation of DNA/RNA/Proteins on polyacrylamide or agarose gels after electrophoresis. The system generally consists of UV light transilluminator, darkroom that block external light and shield user from UV, a computer, software and a CCD camera for image capture.	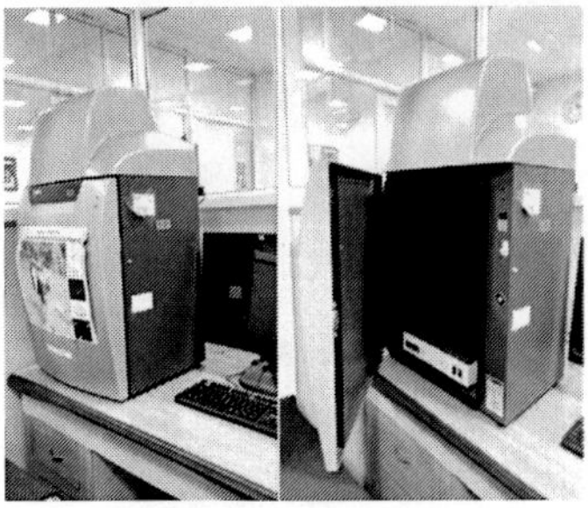 **Fig. 11:** Gel documentation system
Haematology Analyser: An essential equipment for rapidly analysing blood samples to measure parameters such red and white blood cell counts, hemoglobin levels, platelet counts etc., aiding in the diagnosis and monitoring of animal health and diseases.	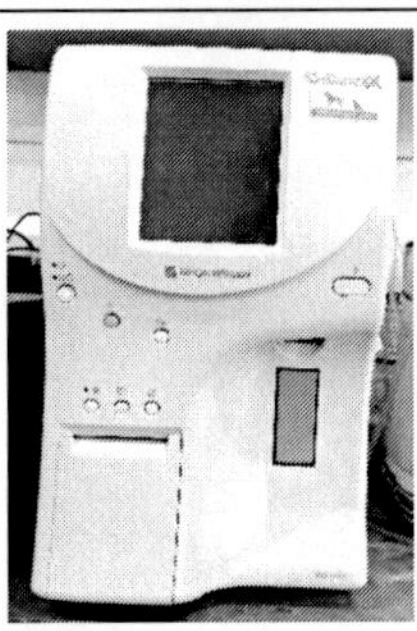 **Fig. 12:** Haematology analyser

Hot Air Oven: To sterilise glassware and instruments (scissors, forceps, scalpels etc.) using dry heat in order to ensure aseptic conditions in the laboratory. They are also used for drying samples and preparing materials for microbiological work.	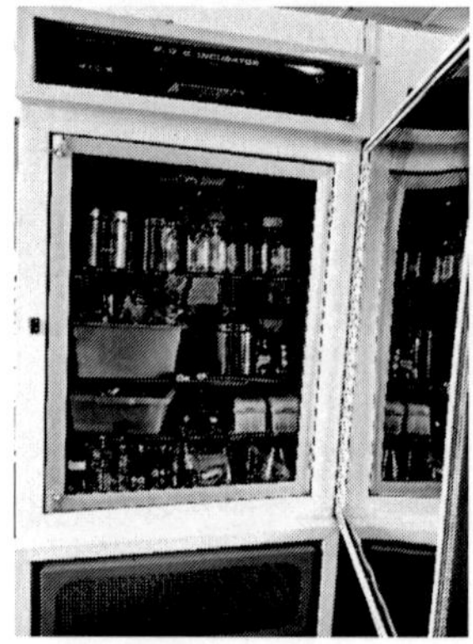 **Fig. 13:** Hot air oven
Incubator: Incubators maintain optimal temperature conditions for culturing microorganisms and cells. The temperature can be set depending on the samples, for example, 37°C for most bacteria cultures, 22-45°C for atypical mycobacteria, 22°C for fungi.	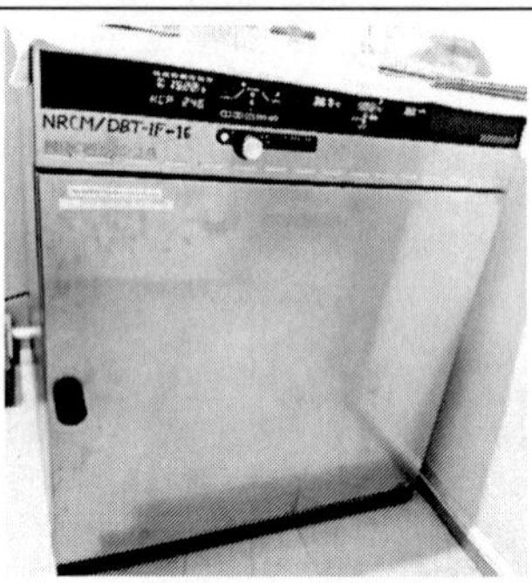 **Fig. 14:** Incubator
Laminar Hood with UV light: Laminar hoods provide a sterile working environment, preventing cross-contamination during sensitive procedures like RNA extraction or tissue culture. The UV light sterilises the workspace, ensuring that experiments remain contamination-free.	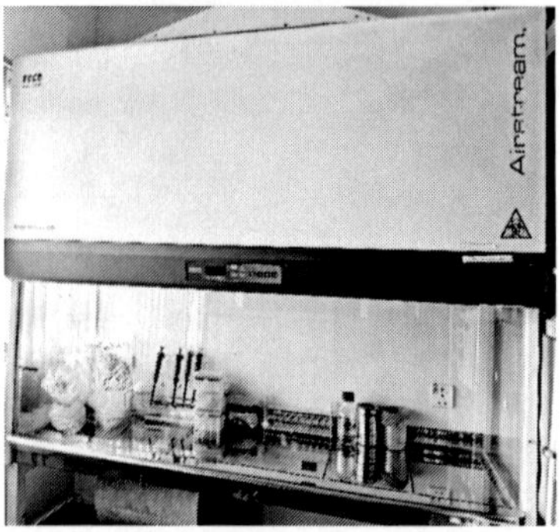 **Fig. 15:** Laminar hood with UV light

Magnetic Stirrer: Magnetic stirrers ensure uniform mixing of solutions, speeding up solute dissolution and reagent preparation. They are widely used for preparing culture media, dissolving agarose, or mixing chemical solutions for analytical experiments	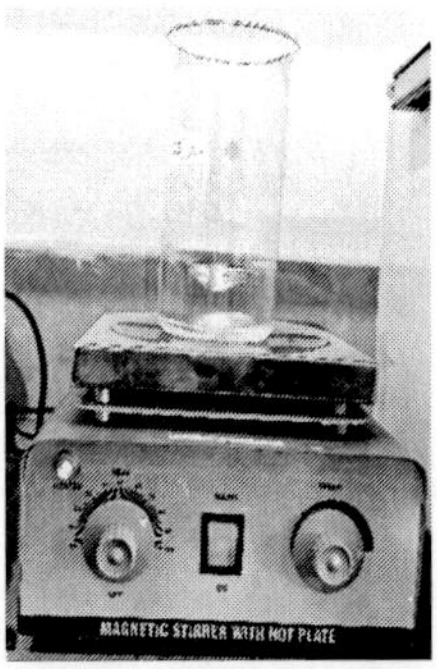 **Fig. 16:** Magnetic stirrer
Micropipette: Micropipettes enable accurate measurement and dispensing of liquid volumes down to microlitres, essential for precision in experimental setups. They are commonly used in molecular biology workflows, such as PCR, where consistency in reagent volumes is critical for reproducibility.	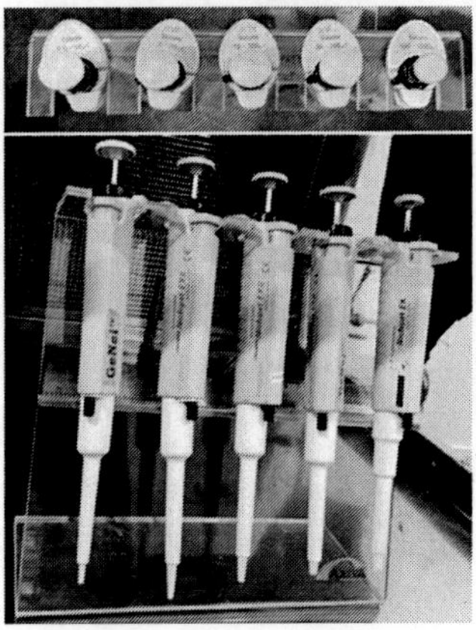 **Fig. 17:** Micropipette
Microscope: A microscope is essential for studying cells, tissues, and parasites. Depending on the goal, stereomicroscopes **(Fig A)** are ideal for examining surface details and larger structures, while fluorescent microscopes **(Fig B)** are used to visualise specific molecules or structures with the help of fluorescent dyes, labeled antibodies, or fluorescent proteins.	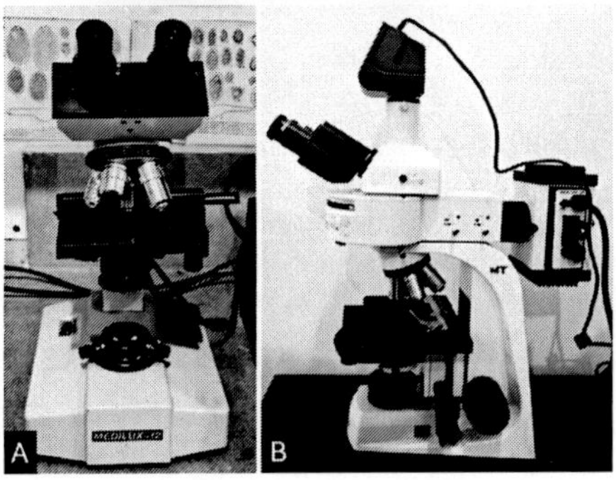 **Fig. 18:** Microscope

Microwave Oven: For quick heating of solutions during routine laboratory works, for example melting of agarose for gel preparation or heating paraffin for histological work.	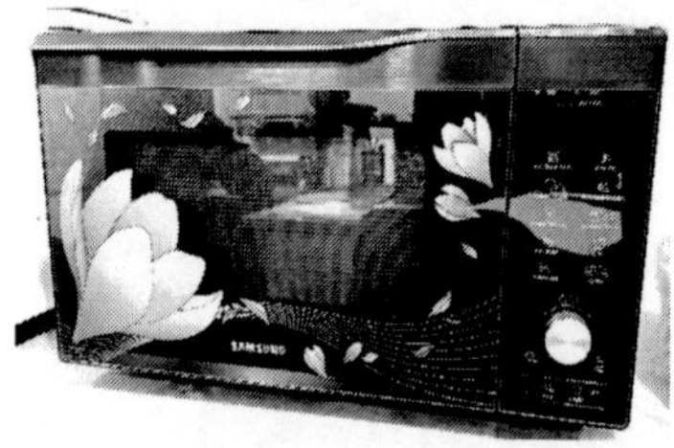 **Fig. 19:** Microwave oven
Multi-channel Pipette: Multichannel pipettes help in simultaneous handling of multiple liquid samples, saving time in high-throughput workflows like ELISA or qPCR. They improve efficiency and consistency and reduce human error that may occur when using single channel pipettes for repetitive pipetting.	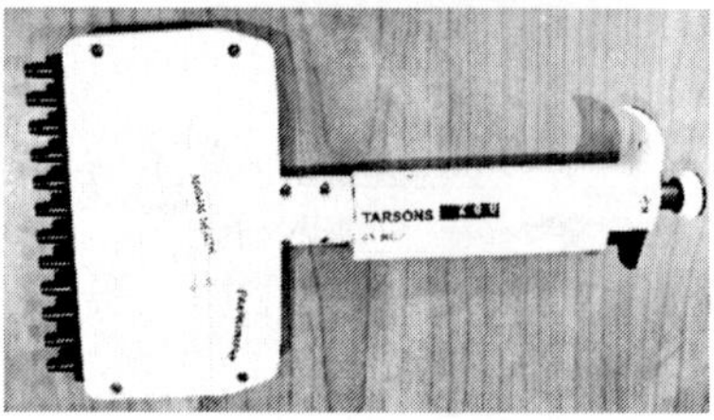 **Fig. 20:** Multi-channel pipette
pH Meter: To measure the pH of various solutions in order to prepare stable reagents and test samples during sensitive assays.	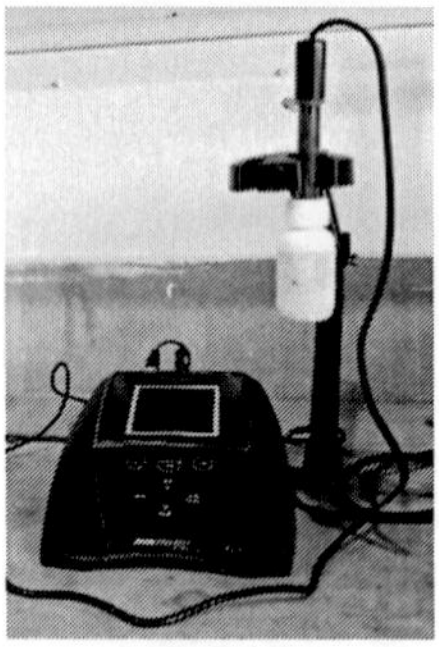 **Fig. 21:** pH meter
Refrigerator: To store the laboratory substances such as media, reagents, and samples at 4–8 °C to ensure stability, viability and functionality for extended periods.	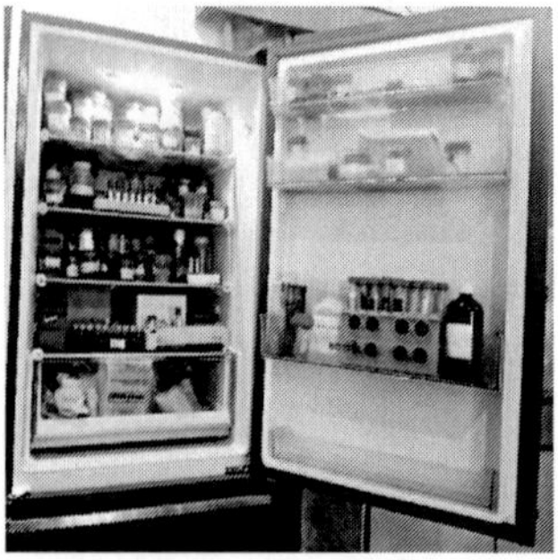 **Fig. 22:** Refrigerator

Thermal cycler: An instrument used for DNA amplification through polymerase chain reaction under precisely controlled temperature and time cycling.	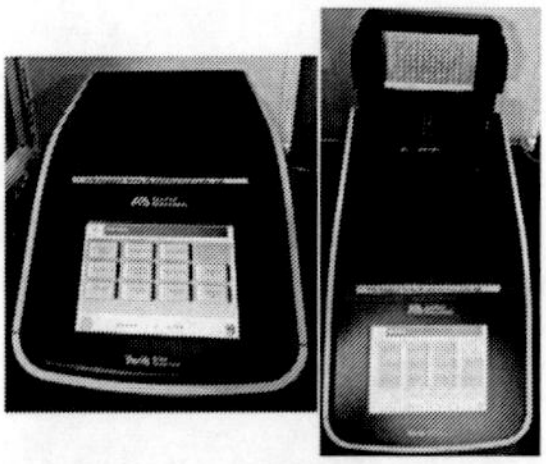 **Fig. 23:** Thermal cycler
UV Spectrophotometer: For quantification of protein, nucleic acids and other molecules by measuring light absorbance. It is essential for assessing DNA/RNA purity, protein concentration and monitoring enzymatic reactions.	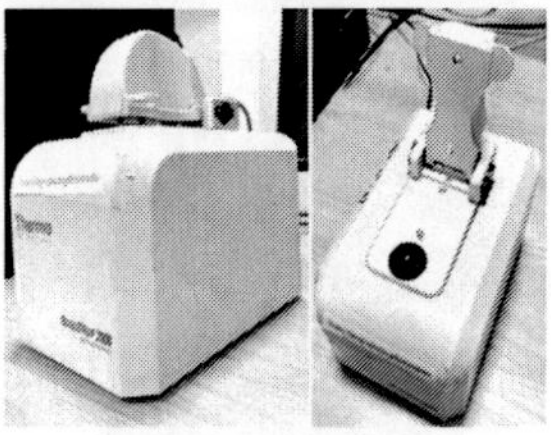 **Fig. 24:** UV spectrophotometer
Vortex Mixer: For rapid and uniform mixing of solutions, homogenisation of reagents and samples. They are widely used for cell resuspensions, mixing PCR reagents or dissolve powders in solutions.	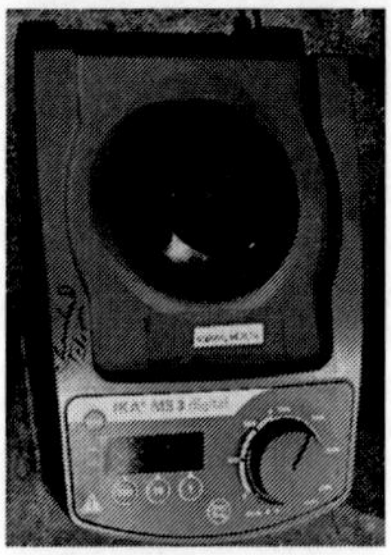 **Fig. 25:** Vortex mixer
Water Bath: For uniform heating of reactants in various reactions such as bacterial assays and enzymatic tests. The uniform heating ensures reproducibility.	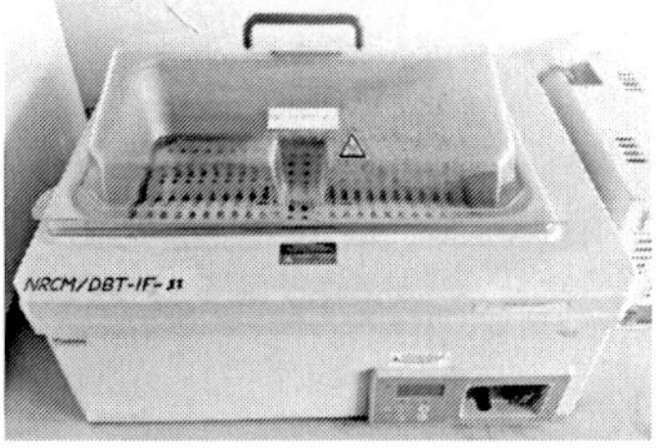 **Fig. 26:** Water bath

Miscellaneous Items

1. Glassware like tissue culture flasks, conical flasks, beakers, centrifuge tubes, syringes, pipettes, glass tubes, scissors, forceps, Tube stands etc.
2. Plastic ware like tissue culture flasks (disposable), petri plates, centrifuge tubes, disposable pipettes, filters, rubber corks/caps, aspiration bulbs, micropipettes, etc.

3. Bunsen burners or alcohol burners
4. Filters like Seitz or Millipore filters, Syringe filters etc.
5. Aprons, gloves, face masks etc.
6. Media and reagents as per requirement.

1.3 Preparation of Solutions and Reagents for Laboratory Use

Please refer to Appendix A.2 for a list of general buffers and reagents, along with their preparation steps.

A variety of solutions and reagents are used in a laboratory. Knowledge about the solutions such as components and concentration, stability, storage, etc. are the key points for its shelf-life and use. Often, the concentrations of solutions are expressed in molarity (pico molar, nano molar, mili molar, etc.) or normality or in percentage. A basic knowledge of analytical chemistry is highly required for the preparation of a solution or reagent.

1.3.1 Preparing Molar Solutions

A molar (M) solution represents the number of moles of solute per liter of solution. To prepare a 1M solution, dissolve the chemical's molecular weight in grams in enough solvent to make 1 liter of solution. For nM solutions, use "n" times the molecular weight.

Solid Chemicals

To prepare molar solutions of solids, simply weigh and dissolve in the appropriate volume of solvent. For example:

1. Preparing 1M NaCl solution:

- Molecular weight of NaCl = 58.5 gm
- Dissolve 58.5 gm NaCl in double distilled water
- Add water until total volume reaches 1000 mL

2. Preparing 0.5M NaCl solution

- Required amount = 0.5 × 58.5 gm (Mol. Weight of NaCl) = 29.25 gm
- Dissolve 29.25 gm NaCl in double distilled water
- Add water until total volume reaches 1000 mL

Liquid Chemicals

For liquids, we must account for density to determine the volume needed. For example:

Preparing 1M acetic acid solution:

Molecular weight of acetic acid = 60.05 gm

Density = 1.049g/mL

$$\text{Required volume} = \frac{\text{Mass}}{\text{Density}} = \frac{60.5}{1.049} = 57.24\text{ml}$$

Therefore, to prepare a 1M solution, add 57.24mL acetic acid to 942.76mL water (total = 1000mL) and mix well.

Safety Note: Always add acid to water, never water to acid, as this can generate excessive heat and potentially cause explosions and acid splashes.

1.3.2 Solution Dilution

To dilute solutions, use the formula: $N_1V_1 = N_2V_2$

Where:

N_1 = Initial concentration

V_1 = Volume of stock solution needed

N_2 = Desired final concentration

V_2 = Desired final volume

Example calculations

1. Diluting formalin from 40% to 10%:

We want: 5 liters of 10% solution

We have: 40% stock solution

$$V_1 = \frac{(N_2V_2)}{N_1} = \frac{(10\% \times 5L)}{40\%} = 1.25L$$

Hence, mix 1.25L of 40% stock with 3.75L water

2. Diluting NaCl from 1M to 10mM:

We want: 50mL of 10mM solution

We have: 1M (1000mM) stock solution

$$V_1 = \frac{(10mM \times 50mL)}{100mM} = 0.5mL$$

Hence, mix 0.5mL of 1M stock with 49.5mL water

1.3.3 Preparing Percent Solutions

Mass percent and volume percent are two ways to express solution concentration:

Mass Percent

The mass percent of a solution is the ratio of the solute mass to the total solution mass, multiplied by 100%:

$$\text{Mass percent} = \left(\frac{\text{Mass of solute}}{\text{Total mass of solution}}\right) \times 100\%$$

Example calculation

If you dissolve 20 gm of salt in 180g of water:

Mass of solute (salt) = 20g

Total mass of solution = 20g + 180g = 200g

$$\text{Mass percent} = \left(\frac{20\text{g}}{200\text{g}}\right) \times 100\% = 10\%$$

This means the solution is 10% salt by mass.

Volume Percent

The volume percent of a solution is the ratio of the solute volume to the total solution volume, multiplied by 100%:

$$\text{Volume percent} = \left(\frac{\text{Volume of solute}}{\text{Volume of solution}}\right) \times 100$$

Example calculation

If you mix 15mL of ethanol with 85mL of water:

Volume of solute (ethanol) = 15mL

Total volume of solution = 15mL + 85mL = 100mL

$$\text{Volume percent} = \left(\frac{15}{100}\right) \times 100 = 15$$

This means the solution is 15% ethanol by volume.

Key differences

- Mass percent is typically used for solid solutes (like salt in water)
- Volume percent is typically used for liquid solutions (like mixing two liquids)
- Mass percent requires weighing ingredients
- Volume percent requires measuring volumes

Note: When mixing liquids, the final volume may not always equal the sum of individual volumes due to molecular interactions, but this simple addition is used for basic calculations.

2

Veterinary Parasitology Techniques

This chapter explores the essential techniques used in veterinary parasitology to collect, identify, and diagnose parasitic infections. These methods are crucial for understanding general animal health, the complex relationships between parasites and their hosts and for tracking disease outbreaks, that will ultimately allow the development of effective control strategies. Whether in a research lab or a clinical setting, the techniques discussed here are widely used to detect and study parasites that impact both domestic and wild animals.

2.1 Collection of Specimens for Parasitological Examinations

Different species of parasites affects almost all parts of the host. These organisms can inhabit virtually every organ system of the host animal, from the brain and lungs to the digestive tract and skin. Therefore, a thorough examination of both living animals and post-mortem cases is essential for collecting parasites and determining cause of death (when applicable). When collecting from live animals, samples should be collected after through exanimation of the animals and following the standard procedure. The collection of correct samples, use of appropriate transport media and proper handling of specimens are crucial factors that directly influence diagnostic accuracy.

The type of specimen collected depends on the methods of identification and diagnosis. For example, diagnosis of blood parasites requires specific types of samples: peripheral blood smears for microscopic examination of hemoprotozoans, serum or plasma for ELISA and other serological tests, and unclotted whole blood for molecular diagnostic methods such as PCR and qPCR.

Further, we must consider not only the location of the parasite within the host but also its life cycle stage and the most appropriate diagnostic methods. For example, some parasites may be detected through simple fecal examination, while others require molecular or serological testing. The success of diagnosis heavily depends on proper specimen collection, appropriate preservation, and careful transport to the laboratory.

The following table (Table 1) outlines major parasitic diseases of veterinary importance, particularly those affecting livestock and large animals. For each disease, specific sampling methods and appropriate collection media have been identified to ensure optimal diagnostic results. The recommendations take into account both the parasite's location within the host and the requirements of various diagnostic techniques, from traditional microscopy to advanced molecular methods.

Table 1: Major parasitic diseases and method for sample collection for diagnostic purposes

Disease	Samples and medium of collection
Gastrointestinal Helminthosis	Fecal samples in sterile container Serum sample for serological investigation.
Bovine Trichomoniosis	Paired serum samples of dam. Preputial washing with NSS/PBS. Vaginal discharges in sterile vials. Tissues of placenta, foetal liver, stomach, kidney in 10% formal saline.
Babesiosis	Blood sample in EDTA & it can be directly used for smear examination. Serum sample for serological examination.
Theileriosis	Serum sample. Peripheral lymph node biopsy/aspirate. Blood sample in EDTA.
Trypanosomiosis	Blood smear (thick and thin). Smear of tissue fluids. Serum sample.
Ectoparatiste	Ectoparasites (ticks, lice, mites, flies etc) in 10 % formalin or 70% alcohol. Skin scrapping in 10% KOH Solution.
Nasal Schistosomiosis	Nasal scrapping/wash in 10% NaOH solution
Microfilarial Disease	Blood sample in EDTA. Tissue sample in 10 % formalin

2.1.1 General Guidelines for Veterinary Specimen Collection

Please refer to Appendix B1 for essential equipment and supplies checklist for sample collection

Pre-Collection Assessment

Review the animal's clinical history thoroughly, including, previous parasitic infections, grazing history and management practices, recent changes in behaviour or productivity and current or recent treatments administered. Note down body condition, hydration status, mucous membrane colour. lymph node enlargement and presence of visible parasites.

Safety Considerations for Large Animal Handling

Animal Restraint

Ensure proper restraining facilities are available (e.g., Travis). Use appropriate sedation when necessary, considering the animal's size and temperament. Have sufficient trained personnel present for safe handling.

Personal Protection

Wear appropriate protective clothing (coveralls, boots), disposable gloves for each animal. Wear face protection when collecting samples that might splash and use arm-length gloves for rectal examination and sampling.

Sample Collection Procedures

Equipment Preparation

- Organise all necessary collection materials before restraining the animal
- Label containers before collecting samples
- Have ice packs or cooling equipment ready if required
- Ensure adequate quantities of preservatives and transport media

Cross Contamination Prevention

- Change gloves between animals
- Use sterile equipment for each sample
- Clean and disinfect any reusable equipment between animals

Packaging and Transport Guidelines

Please refer to Appendix B2 for detailed information to be included along with sample to be sent for laboratory analysis.

Sample packaging

- Use break resistant containers for all specimens
- Ensure screwcap tubes are properly sealed – for long distance shipment, ensure tubes are also sealed with parafilm
- Use appropriate container size for the sample volume
- Select containers with wide mouths for solid specimens
- Package different types of specimens separately
- Use individual sealed bags for each container
- Include absorbent material in case of leakage
- Maintain appropriate temperature conditions

Transport Preparation

- Describe the clinical signs, lesions, tentative diagnosis and treatment given to animal in the letter accompanying the sample to be shipped to the laboratory. Also mention the type of test required as per the tentative diagnosis.
- Mark the parcel 'Biological Material', 'Handle with care', 'Glass material', 'Fragile' etc. in order to avoid damage.
- Keep one copy of covering letter inside sealed plastic bag inside the parcel and send another copy by hand or post separately
- Use insulated containers for temperature sensitive samples
- Include sufficient ice packs or dry ice as needed
- Consider shipping time when selecting preservation methods

2.2 Routine Blood Examination

Routine blood examinations are fundamental diagnostic tools in veterinary medicine that provide crucial information about an animal's health status, disease conditions, and treatment responses. These tests can be broadly categorised into quantitative measurements of various blood components and microscopic examinations. Hematological parameters assess the blood's cellular components and their characteristics, while serum biochemical estimations evaluate organ function, metabolic status, and systemic conditions. Some tests require anticoagulated whole blood to maintain cellular integrity, while others utilise serum obtained after blood clotting for analysing non-cellular components. Microscopic examination includes wet mounts for detecting blood parasites, and thin or thick blood smears for cellular morphology and differential counting. The following sections provide a brief description and protocol of various blood tests that can be done to assess animal health.

Note: please refer to Appendix B4 for troubleshooting blood sample collection issues.

Collection of Whole Blood

Requirements: Syringes, needles, 70% alcohol, scissors, anticoagulants, glass slides, blood collection vials, cotton etc.

Anticoagulants: Commonly used anticoagulants

EDTA (K or Na salt): 1-2 mg/ml of blood (>2mg/ml causes shrinking of cells)

Recommended for routine hematology (best if used within 6 hours)

Heparin: 1-2 mg (0.2 ml of 1 % solution) per ml of blood

Table 2: Sites for blood collection in different species

Site	Species
Jugular Vein	Bovines, equines, sheep and goat and occasionally from dog and cat
Cephalic Vein	Dogs and cats
Sephanous Vein (Hind limb)	Dogs
Anterior Vena cava and Ear Vein	Pigs
Marginal Ear Vein	Cats, small dogs, pigs, rabbits, elephant
Heart	All animals but generally used in small animals.
Wing Vein, Jugular Vein	Poultry
Coccygeal Vein	Rats and mice
Toenail	Pups
Milk Vein	Cattle

- For routine hematology 2 to 5 ml blood is needed from small and large animals, respectively.
- Restrain the animal, clip the hair at the site and apply alcohol or tincture of iodine.
- Insert the dry needle with syringe in the vein and collect the blood using minimum suction, transfer blood immediately into the container with adequate anticoagulant. Gently flip the tube 1-2 times.

Collection of Serum

Serum is the clear, straw-colored fluid obtained after blood clotting and centrifugation, containing proteins, enzymes, hormones, and other soluble components essential for biochemical analysis. It serves as the primary sample type for most biochemical tests and provides valuable diagnostic information about organ function and metabolic disorders. Good quality serum is a must for laboratory investigation of various disease conditions.

1. Collect blood from fasting animals (10 ml from large and 3-5 ml from small animals) in sterile tubes, ideally vacutainer with clotting factors.
2. Avoid multiple needle passage as it causes hemolysis due to mixing with tissue fluid.
3. Keep the tubes in slanting position and allow to clot at room temperature (protect from direct sunlight).
4. After 2-4 hours the serum gets separated from the clotted blood due to the contraction of clot.
5. Transfer the serum tubes to refrigerator (4-6°C). If sample can be delivered with refrigeration within 48 hours to the laboratory then do not

separate serum in the field condition but if it cannot reach the laboratory within 48 hours, then decant the serum into sterile vials.

6. If there is no refrigeration facility, add few drops of 0.2 ml solution of 50,000 units of penicillin and streptomycin per 10 ml of serum to avoid contamination.
7. Do not use merthiolate, fluoride or boric acid in serum if used for living systems, i.e. for experimental inoculation in laboratory animals.
8. If received in the laboratory with the clotted blood in tube, then centrifuge the blood for 15 minutes at 1500 rpm and decant the serum in a sterile vial with pipette.
9. Mishandling, poorly balanced centrifuge or delayed separation of serum from the clot may cause hemolysis of the RBCs thereby affecting the quality of serum.

2.2.1 Hematocrit or Packed Cell Volume (PCV)

This measurement represents the volume percentage of red blood cells in whole blood and provides preliminary information on anemia, dehydration, and polycythemia in animals. It provides rapid, reliable information about an animal's oxygen-carrying capacity and hydration status.

Materials required: Wintrobe tube, PCV tube filler (Pasteur pipette or long needle attached with syringe), Centrifuge machine, Anti coagulated blood sample.

Methods

- Fill Wintrobe tube by inserting the filler into the tube touching to the bottom and pushing the blood and gradually withdrawing the filler inside the tube to the top 10 mark.
- Place Wintrobe tube in a centrifuge with proper balancing and rotate it at 3000 to 4000 rpm for 30 to 45 min.
- Measure the thickness of separated blood elements, observe colour of plasma and calculate PCV.
- PCV (%) = height of red cells in mm / total height of column (mm) x 100
- The intracellular blood protozoan can be demonstrated easily when a slide smear is made and stained from beneath the buffy coat, on top of the red cell column.

Interpretation

- Roughly normal range of PCV = normal range of hemoglobin x 3 for all species.

- Rough RBC count (million / cubic mm of blood) = PCV / 6.
- If PCV < minimum normal range, anemia exists while if PCV > maximum range, hemo-concentration is indicated.
- Buffy coat less than 0.5 mm suggest leukopenia and above 1.5 mm leukocytosis.
- Turbid plasma indicates lipemia. White opaque layer at top of hematocrit indicates hemoglobinemia.

2.2.2 Erythrocyte Sedimentation Rate (ESR)

ESR measures the rate at which red blood cells settle in anticoagulated blood over a specific time period, serving as a non-specific indicator of inflammation and certain disease conditions in animals. It is inversely proportional to the number of red blood cells. The fall of red blood cells is measured in mm in wintrobe tube after intervals 30 minutes, 1 hour, 2 hours and 3 hours.

Materials required: Wintrobe sedimentation tube, tube filler, tube stand, cotton, anticoagulated blood sample.

Method

- Fill the tube with blood up to the '0' mark and put vertically into tube stand.
- Measure fall of erythrocytes (mm) after 30 minutes,1 hour and so on.

Interpretation: An increase in ESR occurs due to increase in plasma proteins in inflammatory conditions and also in hypercholesterolemia and anemia.

Increased ESR is observed in diseases conditions like canine distemper, ICH, leptospirosis, interstitial nephritis, neoplasm and inflammatory conditions like pyometra, pneumonia, pleuritis, peritonitis etc.

2.2.3 Total Leucocytes Count (TLC)

This parameter quantifies the total number of white blood cells present in a blood sample, providing information about infection, inflammation, stress, and immune system status in animals. Changes in TLC can indicate various pathological conditions.

Materials required: Hemocytometer, WBC diluting fluid, diluting pipette for WBCs (white bead), Distilled water, Alcohol, Acetone, etc.

Procedure

- Suck blood in WBC pipette up to 0.5 mark and then add diluting fluid exactly up to 11 mark (blood dilution 1:20).
- Rotate the pipette between palms for proper mixing of the content.

- Discard first few drops of fluid and charge the chamber in hemocytometer after putting a cover slip over platform and observe under low power (10x objective) of microscope.
- Count WBCs in 4 primary squares.
- TLC (leucocyte/microliter) = total no. of leucocytes (all 4 primary squares) ×50.

2.2.4 Total Erythrocyte Count (TEC)

TEC measures the total number of red blood cells per unit volume of blood, helping evaluate an animal's oxygen-carrying capacity and diagnose conditions affecting red blood cell production or destruction. It is useful for classifying types of anemia.

Materials required: Haemocytometer, RBCs diluting fluid, pipette for RBCs (red bead), Distilled water, Alcohol, Acetone etc.

Erythrocyte Diluting Fluid

1. Normal salt solution (0.85 g NaCl in 100 ml distilled water)
2. Gower's Solution: Anhydrous sodium sulfate (12.5 g) and glacial Acetate (33.3 ml) in 200 ml of distilled water.

Procedure

- Suck blood in RBCs diluting pipette up to 0.5 marks and then add RBC diluting fluid exactly up to 101 marks (blood dilution 1:200).
- Rotate the pipette between palms for proper mixing of the content.
- Discard the first few drops of fluid and charge the chamber after putting a cover slip over platform and see under low power (10x objective) of microscope.
- Count 4 secondary squares and one central secondary square.
- TEC = Total no. of erythrocytes (all 5 secondary squares) x 10,000 = total erythrocyte/microlitre.

2.2.5 Differential Leucocytes Count (DLC)

This test determines the relative percentages of different types of white blood cells. When blood is spread on a slide, neutrophils rush to the edge of the film, lymphocytes remain in the body of smear, while monocytes and eosinophils tend to become evenly distributed throughout. Avoid thick and tail ends of the smear for counting. Examine edge of the smear for intracellular parasites.

Materials required: Glass slides, stains (Leishman's stain/modified Wright's stain/Giemsa's stain)

Methods of counting cells: Straight edge method, cross sectional method, Battlement method

Procedure

- Stain the thin blood smear slide with suitable stain (Leishman's stain/ modified Wright's stain/Giemsa's stain).
- Examine the blood smear under oil immersion and count at least 100 leucocytes (neutrophils, eosinophils, basophils, lymphocytes and monocytes), including immature neutrophils using DLC counter or by tally method.
- Absolute count is derived as type of cell/100 x TLC

Factors influencing DLC

- Age (calf in 1st week -low levels of lymphocytes and higher neutrophils, swine at birth 70% neutrophils, young dog more lymphocytes).
- Animal species like cattle, sheep, goat and pig lymphocytes are always in higher concentration compared to other WBC.
- Exercise (neutrophilia), emotional state (neutrophilia in fear).

Shift to left: Excess number of young forms of the granulocytic series cells in peripheral circulation

- *Regenerative shift to left:* TLC elevated above normal, and this is associated with the occurrence of immature forms of neutrophils in the peripheral circulation.
- *Degenerative shift to left:* TLC is normal or below normal, associated with occurrence of below normal number of mature neutrophils and the presence of immature neutrophils, many of which show toxic changes.

Shift to right: Abnormal number of hyper segmented neutrophils or aged cells.

2.2.6 Eosinophil Count (EC)

Eosinophil counts specifically measure this type of white blood cell, which typically increases in parasitic infections and allergic conditions in animals. Monitoring eosinophil levels is particularly important in veterinary medicine due to the frequency of parasitic infections.

Materials required: WBCs diluting pipette, hemocytometer, propylene glycol fluid.

Procedure

- Draw blood to 0.5 mark of the WBC diluting pipette.
- Suck propylene glycol fluid up to 11 mark and mix well for 2 minutes.
- Fill the hemocytometer chamber for counting and wait for 15 minutes for complete lysing of RBCs.

- Count eosinophils in all 9 (4+5) squares of each chamber.
- Average eosinophils/chamber X 11.1= number/cmm of blood.

2.2.7 Platelets Count

Platelet count is performed to evaluate the number of platelets per microliter of blood, aiding in the diagnosis of bleeding disorders, infections, or inflammatory conditions in animals.

Materials required: RBCs diluting pipette, hemocytometer, Rees-Ecker solution.

Rees-Ecker solution

- Sodium citrate: 3.8 g
- Formaldehyde, 40%: 0.2 ml
- Brilliant cresyl blue: 0.1 g
- Distilled water: 100 ml

Keep stoppered and in refrigerator. Filter before use.

Procedure

- Draw the blood into erythrocyte diluting pipette up to 0.5 mark.
- Draw the platelet diluting fluid (Rees-Ecker) to the 101 mark.
- Mix thoroughly for 5 minutes, discard first few drops.
- Fill both the chambers of hemocytometer.
- Keep the chamber in a moist covered petri dish for 15 minutes to settle the cells.
- Count the thrombocytes in the entire central grid area on both sides of hemocytometer.
- Calculate the total number of thrombocytes x 1000 = no. thrombocytes/μl.

2.2.8 Hemoglobin Estimation

Hemoglobin concentration indicates the oxygen-carrying capacity of blood and is essential for diagnosing and classifying various types of anemia in animals. It directly correlates with the animal's ability to transport oxygen to tissues. Hemoglobin is found in saturated state in RBCs. The iron content is 0.335% or 3.35 mg/gm of Hb and oxygen carrying capacity is 1.36 cc/gm of Hb.

Acid Hematin method

RBCs treated with N/10 HCl acid form brown color acid hematin, which is matched with color standard.

Materials required: Sahli's hemoglobinometer, N/10 HCl (1 ml of conc. HCL in 99 ml of DWW), distilled water, blood samples and cotton, etc.

Procedure

- Take 5-6 drops N/10 HCl in graduated tube (avoid too much acid).
- Add properly mixed blood with measuring pipette up to the mark.
- Mix the contents with glass rod and add small amount of NSS or N/10 HCl along with mixing till the brown color matches with standard (do not keep blood and acid mixture for a long time).
- Reading is made in gm/100 ml of blood

Cyanmethaemoglobin method

The haemoglobin is converted to a cyanmethaemoglobin with cyanide present in the diluting solution which is read as OD value indicating Hb concentration.

Material required: Drabkin's diluent solution [Mix sodium bicarbonate (1.0 g), potassium cyanide (50 mg), potassium ferricyanide $K_3Fe(CN)6$ (200 mg) in 1000 ml of distilled water and store in brown bottle at 4 °C] and colorimeter.

Procedure: Take 5 ml Drabkin's diluent solution in a colorimeter cuvette, add 0.02 ml of blood and mix thoroughly and let stand for 10 minutes before reading OD at 540 nm against a blank of either Drabkin's solution or distilled water.

Interpretation: Decrease in Hb content reveals anemia due to hemorrhage, parasitism (hemonchosis), ticks, lice, infectious and non-infectious diseases, protozoan diseases, leptospirosis, bacillary haemoglobinuria, poisoning by onion, cruciferous plants, nutritional deficiency (Cu and Cobalt), chronic suppurative process, etc.

Table 3: Normal blood values in different animals

Species	Erythro. (10^6)	Leuko. (10^3)	Hb (g/dl)	PCV (%)	Neut. (%)	Lympho. (%)	Mono. (%)	Eosino. (%)
Cattle	6-8	7-8	8-14	30-50	20-40	40-70	3-15	1-15
Sheep	8-10	7-8	10-14	30-50	20-40	40-70	1-12	1-10
Goat	12-15	5-13	8-14	30-40	20-40	50-70	1-4	3-8
Pig	5-8	8-20	10-16	30-50	30-50	40-60	1-10	1-11
Dog	5-8	8-12	11-15	40-60	60-80	10-30	2-10	2-10
Cat	5-9	8-15	8-15	30-40	60-70	20-40	1-7	2-10
Horse	7-13	5-13	10-18	30-60	50-65	20-40	2-10	2-10
Mithun	6-8	7-12	10-12	30-45	30-60	35-70	2-7	2-5

2.2.9 Blood Examination for Detection of Microfilaria

The Knott's method is a widely used diagnostic technique for the detection and concentration of microfilariae in blood samples. It is particularly useful in veterinary diagnostics for detecting microfilarial infections in animals, such as those caused by *Dirofilaria* species.

Knott's method

1. Collect peripheral blood, preferably during the evening or at the peak of the animal's body temperature.
2. Take 1 ml of whole blood in a centrifuge tube.
3. Dilute it with 9 ml of 2 % formalin (1: 9 v/v)
4. Centrifuge for 5 minutes at 3000 rpm.
5. Discard the supernatant.
6. Then mix the sediment thoroughly with a drop of 0.1% methylene blue or 0.2% methyl green solution by a pipette.
7. Transfer a small amount of the sediment to a clean microscopic slide.
8. Put a cover slip over the preparation.
9. Examine under microscope for microfilaria.

Microfilariae of the pathogenic heartworm *(Dirofilaria immitis)* and of other, less pathogenic filarioid species can be discriminated on the basis of several criteria such as size, morphology, movement, numbers, staining characteristics; this needs experience, knowledge of regional prevalence, and thus it should best be performed by an expert diagnostic unit.

Microfilaria of *D. reconditum* tend to move rapidly across the microscopic field with a snake like movement. *D. immitis* microfilaria tend to remain in the general area and coil and uncoil.

Table 4: Morphological features of filarial parasites

Morphology	*Dirofilaria immitis*	*Dipetalonema reconditum*
Body shape	Usually straight	Usually curved
Body length	295-325 um	250-288 um
Midbody width	5-7.5 um	4.5-5.5 um
Shape of cranial end	Tapered	Blunt
Shape of tail	Straight	Usually curved or hooked

2.2.10 Best Practices and Techniques for Routine Blood Examination

- Always collect blood samples before feeding or medication
- Use appropriate anticoagulants based on the intended tests:

  - EDTA for complete blood counts
  - Heparin for biochemical tests
  - Clot-activator tubes for serum collection
- Fill collection tubes to the correct mark to maintain proper blood-to-anticoagulant ratio
- Mix samples gently by inverting 2-3 times immediately after collection
- Process samples within recommended timeframes
- Complete blood count: within 4 hours
- ESR: within 2 hours
- Serum separation: allow up to 1 hour for clotting

2.3 Staining of Films and Smears on Glass Slides

The visualisation and identification of microorganisms, cells, and their components in veterinary diagnostics relies on various staining techniques. Different cellular constituents in films and smears exhibit specific affinities for different stains, similar to their behavior in tissue sections. Basic dyes are predominantly employed, often enhanced through mordants (such as phenol or weak alkalis), heat application, or extended staining duration. While simple stains like methylene blue and polychrome methylene blue provide basic information about cellular morphology and presence of organisms, differential and special stains offer more detailed insights into specific cellular components and microorganisms. The Romanowsky stain, which was originally developed for the visualisation of blood cells and parasites, has since been improved and incorporated into more refined staining techniques such as Leishmann, Giemsa, and others. These stains are particularly effective in differentiating various types of blood cells and detecting intracellular pathogens like protozoa, bacteria, and filarial parasites.

Fixation and preparation of blood samples

- In order to ensure glass slides are grease free, wash the glass slides with soft soap and rinse with distilled water. Then, dip the slides in isopropyl or 95% alcohol and dry using soft clean cloth to the slides.
- Take a grease free slide (say slide A) in left hand.
- Put a small drop of blood on narrow side of slide A (held towards middle finger).
- Take another slide (say slide B) in right hand and put its lower long edge on slide A.

- Form 30-40° angle between slide A and B with lower edge of slide B in forward direction.
- First move the edge of slide B in backward direction to touch the blood drop and continue so that blood spread along the edge of slide B.
- Now move the slide B in forward direction in single stroke (continuous).
- Fast dry the slide by waving in air to avoid crenation of erythrocytes.
- A well-prepared blood film is seen smooth in appearance without any holes or waves.
- Stain blood film within 24 hours for best results.

Fixation and preparation of other samples

- Clean glass slides thoroughly to ensure they are grease-free by washing with soft soap, rinsing with distilled water, treating with isopropyl or 95% alcohol, and drying with a clean soft cloth.
- For liquid samples (exudates and other bodily fluids), place approximately 20 μL of the sample on a clean slide.
- Use the same two-slide technique as blood smears - place the spreading slide at a 30-40° angle and create the smear as described in the blood smear protocol.
- For fecal samples, first create a thin suspension by mixing a small amount of faeces with physiological saline directly on the slide, then spread using the two-slide technique, adjusting the angle if needed for proper spreading.
- Unlike blood smears which can be air-dried, these samples require immediate fixation to prevent cellular degradation.
- Fix the slides immediately after spreading by either:
  - Immersing in 95% methanol for 3-5 minutes, or
  - Using a methanol-based spray fixative
- Allow the fixed slides to dry completely before proceeding with staining.
- For optimal results, stain the fixed slides within 24 hours, though properly fixed slides can be stored for longer periods if necessary.
- Check that the final preparation appears smooth and evenly spread, without clumps or gaps in the sample.

Please refer to Appendix B5 for issues and troubleshooting for the following staining methods

2.3.1 Leishman's Staining

A Romanowsky-type stain that differentiates blood cells and blood parasites, Leishman stain is valuable technique in veterinary hematology for its ability to clearly demonstrate nuclear and cytoplasmic details. It is especially useful in identifying blood-borne parasites like *Babesia, Theileria, Trypanosoma*, etc., Bacteria, Spirochaetes and Chlamydia.

Solution Composition: Leishman stain power : 0.15 gm
Absolute Methyl Alcohol : 100 ml

Mix it and pour into a dark bottle and keep for a few weeks for maturation prior to use.

Staining protocol

- Cover the blood or tissue smear with Leishman's stain solution for 1 min.
- Dilute the stain with double the volume of distilled water with **slightly acidic pH (6.5)** or tap water if the water is not very hard.
- Mix by pipetting up and down.
- Allow the smear to stain for 20 min, wash off the stain with tap water, and blot it dry.
- Observe under the microscope using oil immersion objective.

Interpretation: The procedure is very useful for examining blood smears and to detect haemoprotozoans and other micro-organisms such as *Pasteurella* organisms, chlamydial inclusion bodies, haemophilus, and spirochaetes.

2.3.2 Ziehl -Neelsen staining

The Ziehl-Neelsen (Z-N) staining method relies on the unique cell wall characteristics of acid-fast bacteria, particularly *Mycobacterium* species. The primary stain, carbol fuchsin, contains phenol which acts as a mordant to enhance stain penetration. When heat is applied during staining, it melts the waxy lipids in the bacterial cell wall and facilitates the entry of the dye-phenol complex into the cell. Once stained, the mycobacteria retain the bright red carbol fuchsin even when exposed to strong acid decolorisers like hydrochloric acid, hence the term "acid-fast". A contrasting counterstain (typically methylene blue or malachite green) is then applied to provide background differentiation, making the red acid-fast bacteria clearly visible against the blue or green background.

An important point to remember is that, environmental mycobacteria found in tap water, which also contain lipid-rich cell walls, can produce false-positive results, appearing as clustered red bacilli at various focal planes. Thus, to ensure reliable results, each staining procedure should include a positive control specimen, as carbol fuchsin's staining efficiency can deteriorate over time, and newly prepared solutions may not always function optimally.

Fixation and preparation of sample

- Prepare thin smear from clinical samples (faeces, nasal washing, sputum, rectal pinch, biopsy, body fluid etc).
- Prepare fecal smear directly/by taking in a muslin cloth or by using sediments after decantation (1 gm faeces in 10 ml DW) and centrifugation for 20 minutes@ 4000g. It is more sensitive than direct smear method.
- From tubercle nodule prepare smear from the periphery of the lesion since the necrotic centre usually contains fewer viable organisms.
- Suspected exudates for TB are treated with 4% NaOH as decontaminant before centrifuging the suspension for concentration and smear is prepared with the sediment.
- Heat fix the smear over flame avoiding too much heating (should be bearable on skin).

Solution Composition

Carbol fuchsin	Basic fuchsin	:	02 gm
	Absolute alcohol	:	10 ml
	Solution of phenol (1: 20) or crystals	:	100 ml, 5 gm
	Distilled water	:	100 ml
Decolouriser	Hydrochloric acid	:	2 ml
	Ethanol	:	98 ml
Malachite green	Malachite green	:	0.3 gm
	Distilled water	:	100 ml

An alternative and quicker preparation is as

Basic fuchsin (Powder)	:	05 gm
Phenol (Crystal)	:	25 gm
Alcohol (95% or absolute)	:	50 ml
Distilled water	:	500 ml

Staining protocol for Tuberculosis and Para Tuberculosis

- Smears should be fixed with heat.
- Flood the smear over slide with carbol fuchsin and heat gently below the slide to steaming for 3 minutes; leave it for 5 minutesto cool.

- Decolorise the smear until thinner parts are decolorised and the heavier portion remains pink.
- Counter stain with 1 % methylene blue or 0.3 % malachite green for 1 minute.
- Wash in water, and blot dry the slide.
- Observe the smear in oil immersion under the microscope.

Interpretation: The acid -fast bacteria (TB and Para TB) are stained red and tissue cells and other bacteria are blue. Each smear or tissue section should be examined for about 45 minutes to declare the results. As per OIE recommendation, presence of 3-4 strongly acid-fast organisms in clusters warrants a diagnosis of paratuberculosis. Presence of AFO in singles only quite similar to the morphology of *Mycobacterium avium subsp. paratuberculosis* should be regarded as doubtful. Smears – especially those made from faeces – may contain saprophytes and other mycobacteria, which should be differentiated from *M.A. paratuberculosis.* Results of microscopic smears examination should also be correlated with clinical signs.

2.3.3 Modified Z-N Technique

An adaptation of the traditional Z-N stain that is optimised for detecting acid-fast organisms such as *Cryptosporidium*, *Isospora*, and *Cyclospora* in fecal samples. This modification uses stronger decolorisation and different timing to better differentiate these parasitic organisms, which appear as bright red spherical structures against a blue-green background. It is particularly useful for identifying enteric parasites that conventional parasitological techniques might have missed.

Protocol

- Air-dry the thin fecal smears on glass slide and pass quickly through a flame to fix it.
- Stain with Ziehl-Neelsen's carbol-fuchsin solution for 2 min.
- Rinse with tap water.
- Rinse for a few seconds with acid alcohol (3% HCl in 70% ethanol).
- Rinse again with tap water.
- Counter stain with Brilliant Green for 2 min.
- Rinse again with tap water.
- Air-dry the slide.

Observe the stained slide under immersion oil objective (100x). Parasites such as *Cryptosporidia*, *Isospora*, and *Cyclospora* appear bright red on a blue-green background.

Alternative method

- Mix a drop of diarrhoeic faeces with equal quantity of carbol-fuchsine on a glass slide and prepare a thin smear.
- After air-drying, examine the slide directly at a magnification of 1000x, using immersion oil.
- The oocysts measure 4-5 µm in diameter and appear as thick-walled, red granules.

2.3.4 Giemsa Staining

This technique is particularly effective for identifying and studying haemoprotozoans such as *Babesia, Theileria*, and *Plasmodium* species in veterinary samples. The stain's combination of azure, eosin, and methylene blue components creates distinct color differentiation that helps visualise nuclear and cytoplasmic details of both parasites and blood cells.

Fixation and preparation of sample: Prepare the thin blood smear as discussed earlier. The smear should be prepared on clean slides, air dried and fixed in absolute methanol for 3-5 min.

Staining solution

Giemsa powder	:	1 g.
Methyl alcohol	:	66 cc
Glycerin	:	66 cc.

Staining Protocol

Rapid Method

- Fix the film in methyl alcohol for 3 min.
- Stain in a mixture of 1 part of stock and 10 parts of buffer (pH 6.8) for 45 minutes to 1 hour or stain with 1 part of stock and 5 parts of buffer for 15-20 min.
- Wash the film with buffer solution and allow differentiating for about half a minute.
- Blot and air-dry the film.

Slow method

- Prepare solution by adding 1 ml of stock stain solution and 20 ml of buffer solution (pH 6.8) in coupling jar and keep the blood film slides for staining overnight.
- Wash with buffer solution till they are differentiated, blot and air-dry.

2.3.5 D' Antoni's Iodine Staining

An iodine-based staining solution specifically designed for rapid visualisation of protozoan trophozoites, cysts, and helminth eggs in fresh fecal samples. This stain temporarily immobilises motile organisms while enhancing the visibility of internal structures and is thus useful for identifying and differentiating various parasitic stages. It is ideal for quick screening of intestinal parasites.

Fixation and preparation of sample: Small portion of faeces mixed with a drop of iodine reagent on a glass slide.

Staining Composition

Potassium iodide	:	1 gm.
Distilled water	:	100 ml
Iodine	:	1.5 gm.

Staining protocol

- Put a small drop of iodine reagent on a glass slide.
- Mix a small portion of the faeces into the solution with a wooden stick.
- Put a cover slip and examine under the microscope, first low magnification then high.

Interpretation: The parasitic ova and cysts take iodine, giving them dark brown color against yellowish background.

2.3.6 Modified Wright's Stain

A specialised blood stain optimised for detecting and studying blood parasites, particularly trypanosomes. This modification provides enhanced contrast for visualising the distinctive morphological features of blood-borne parasites while maintaining excellent differentiation of blood cell components. It is especially useful for identifying flagellated protozoa.

***Fixation and preparation of sample*:** The blood smears or tissue impressions are air dried and stained with the Wright's stain.

Solution Composition

Wright's stain powder	:	300 mg.
Giemsa stain powder	:	30 mg.
Methyl alcohol	:	100 ml.

Staining Protocol

- Cover the unfixed blood film with undiluted stain and allow it to sit for 1 min.

- Add double the volume of buffer solution (pH 6.6) and mix, then allow it to sit for 10 minutes.
- Flood the slide with buffer solution until the film appears bright pink.

Interpretation: The infecting agents appear red in color. Blood cells take red and blue staining of cytoplasm and nucleus respectively.

2.3.7 Lactophenol Cotton Blue Staining

A unique mounting medium combined with a stain that serves multiple purposes in fungal identification. The lactic acid component preserves fungal structures, phenol acts as a killing agent, and cotton blue selectively stains fungal elements blue against a clear background. This combination makes it an essential tool in veterinary mycology for examining and identifying fungal elements while maintaining their structural integrity.

Fixation and preparation of sample: The skin scrapings are mixed with a drop of cotton blue stain.

Solution Composition

Phenol (melted)	:	20 ml
Lactic acid	:	20 ml
Glycerol	:	40 ml
Aniline blue (Water soluble)	:	500 mg

Heat the phenol, lactic acid and glycerol together at 70°C and then add aniline blue.

Staining protocol

- This staining procedure is very useful for the diagnosis of fungal diseases.
- Prepare a smear on a glass slide from the infected tissue.
- Mix a few drops of lactophenol cotton blue stain with the tissue exudate or smear.
- Cover it with cover slip and seal, if need be, with nail polish.
- Examine under microscope at high magnifications.

Interpretation: The fungus takes on a blue color.

2.3.8 Best Practices and Techniques for Sample Staining

1. Quality Control Measures

- Maintain positive control slides for each staining procedure
- Document lot numbers and expiration dates of reagents

- Regular calibration of pH meters and other equipment
- Temperature monitoring of storage conditions

2. Sample Preparation

- Ensure proper thickness of smears/films
- Allow complete air drying before fixation
- Use clean, grease-free slides
- Proper labelling and identification

3. Reagent Maintenance

- Store reagents according to manufacturer recommendations
- Use fresh working solutions
- Regular quality checks of stock solutions
- Proper disposal of expired reagents

4. Environmental Factors

- Maintain proper laboratory temperature (20-25°C)
- Control humidity levels with proper ventilation and dehumidifiers
- Protect light-sensitive reagents
- Use clean, dust-free work area

5. Documentation

- Maintain detailed records of issues and solutions
- Regular review of protocols
- Quality control logs

2.4 Microscopic Examination of Cytological Preparations

Cytological examination is a rapid, cost-effective, and minimally invasive diagnostic tool compared to histological analysis. It serves as an important first-line diagnostic technique in veterinary medicine for evaluating various pathological conditions. This technique allows for immediate assessment of body fluids, lymph nodes, airways, accessible masses, bone marrow, and other tissues in live animals. The diagnostic value of cytology heavily depends on proper sample collection, preparation, and staining techniques. Samples must be properly air-dried and protected from formalin fumes, excessive humidity, or extreme temperatures to maintain cellular integrity.

Table 5: Types of specimens for cytological examination

Type	Specimen
Body Fluid Samples	Pleural and peritoneal fluids Synovial fluid Cerebrospinal fluid (CSF) Bronchoalveolar lavage (BAL) Urine sediment Prostatic wash Vaginal/uterine wash
Tissue Samples	Superficial masses Internal organs Lymph nodes Bone marrow Skin lesions Mammary gland secretions

Materials: Microscope, Slides, Syringe, Needle, Stains etc.

Fixation and preparation of different sample types

Fluid samples

- Collect fluid samples in EDTA tube and process within 30 minutes of collection
- Centrifuge cell poor samples (thin, watery, transparent) at 500-1000 rpm and prepare smear from the sediment.
- Prepare direct smears from cell rich samples

Touch Smear

- Prepared touch smear from ulcerated masses surfaces.
- Take a fine needle aspiration (FNA) from below the superficial aspect of the masses.
- The blood should be wiped off with blotting paper from the surface of masses (spleen, liver) before making the smears.
- Firm masses should be scrapped with scalpel or blade to loosen cells and facilitate exfoliation.

Aspiration

- Use 22 G needle with a 10 ml syringe for suction irrespective of species.
- Aspirate the mass 2-4 times with the syringe plunger and remove the needle.
- Remove the needle from the syringe, fill air in the syringe and push the material over a glass slide to prepare the smear.
- Prepare as many smears as possible from the aspirate

Scraping Technique

- Useful for surface lesions and firm masses
- Use scalpel blade at 90° angle
- Collect material from multiple sites
- Transfer collected material onto slides
- Spread gently without crushing cells

Staining Options

1. Rapid Romanowsky-type Stains

Diff-Quick (most common)

Wright-Giemsa

May-Grünwald Giemsa

Leishman's stain

2. Special Stains

New methylene blue (for blood parasites)

Gram stain (for bacteria)

Acid-fast stains (for mycobacteria)

Sudan stains (for lipids)

Periodic acid Schiff (PAS) for fungi

Papanicolaou stain (for detailed nuclear features)

Staining protocol: As described for blood smears in Section 2.3.

2.5 Identification of Parasites through Fecal Examination and Culture

Please refer to Appendix B3.2 for troubleshooting issues with fecal sample collection

A laboratory unit for routine diagnostic coproscopy can be installed at a reasonable cost and effort. Equipment, material and tools necessary for microscopic fecal examination of specimens from the veterinary practice are as follows

- Plastic specimen containers with tight fitting lid
- Compound microscope (Objectives: 10, 40,100X; eyepiece: 10 X)
- Dissecting microscope and magnifying glass
- Centrifuge machine, Centrifuge tubes (Plastic or glass)
- Slides and Coverslips
- Wooden/ plastic spatulas

- Sieves with different mesh sizes
- Beakers, Petridishes, Pasteur pipettes, Measuring cylinder, Dissection needles, Forceps, Flotation solutions etc.

Collection of Faeces for Examination and Culture

Proper fecal sample collection is necessary for accurate parasitological examination. Samples collected directly from freshly voided faeces or from the rectum of the animal provide the most reliable results for diagnostic purposes.

- Use clean, wide-mouth containers with screw caps for collection
- Always wear disposable gloves during collection
- For small animals, induce defecation by inserting a moistened finger into the rectum and gently massaging until external sphincter relaxes
- Collect samples from multiple animals in affected herds
- Label containers with complete animal details and collection time
- Label the container with the details of the animal.
- Samples should be collected from several animals in affected herds. Fecal samples collected from the ground in a field in which the animal has been running are less useful for diagnostic purposes.

Fecal samples should be examined under microscope (10X and 40X) either simply by making a thin smear of the suspension of the faeces or after subjecting the faeces to concentration methods such as centrifugation and floatation of the faeces.

2.5.1 Direct Examination

It is effective only in cases where the concentration of the eggs is high, and it is frequently difficult to identify the eggs due to the presence of detritus. Further, it gives only qualitative results and no information about the severity of the infestation.

- Prepare an emulsion of the faeces by mixing it with water.
- Take a small drop of the emulsion over a glass slide and spread to form a thin film.
- Examine the film under microscope at low and high power of objective.

2.5.2 Sedimentation Method

It is a commonly used method for examination of helminthes eggs in faeces because due to the sedimentation, most of the eggs get settled as sediment and are easily observed.

- Take 3 g of faeces; mix it with water in a pestle and mortar.
- Strain it with a seive into a glass beaker.
- Allow to settle for 20-30 minutes to sediment under gravity.
- For fast sedimentation, transfer the suspension to centrifuge tubes and centrifuge at 2000 rpm for 2 min.
- Gently discard the supernatant.
- Repeat the washing step for 4-5 times till the supernatant becomes clear.
- Take a drop of sediment to examine under microscope.

2.5.3 Flotation Method

The most effective egg counting methods involve separating eggs from fecal debris by flotation in different solutions. The type of egg recovered depends on the specific gravity of the solution used. Half-saturated NaCl (1.125) can recover *Trichostrongylid* and *Strongylid* eggs, but fully saturated NaCl (1.204) is preferred as a general-purpose solution. For *Fasciola* eggs, saturated $ZnSO_4$ (1.364) is recommended, while saturated MgSOMgSO_4 is suitable for *Metastrongylus* eggs. If the eggs are needed for purposes such as culturing, a saturated sucrose solution is preferable, as it has less impact on egg viability than other solutions. Place a lump of faeces (5-10g or a few fecal pellets (5-10) of sheep or goats) in a beaker.

- Add approximately 50-100 ml of tap water and mix thoroughly with a spatula/rod until all the fecal material are broken down.
- The mixture is poured through a wire mesh seive with an aperture of 500-800 µm to remove large lumps. The strained fluid is caught in a bowl. The seive is rinsed with water and the debris left on the screen is discarded.
- Allow the mixture to stand for 20-30 minutes or centrifuge at 2000 rpm for 2 minutes. Discard the supernatant and mix the sediment with clean tap water. Repeat this step two to three times till the supernatant becomes clear.
- Finally, take the sediment and mix with high density/specific gravity solution. Prepare solutions of different specific gravity i.e. saturated and half saturated solutions of NaCl, $MgSO_4$ and $ZnSO_4$.
- Fill the tubes with high density solutions and leave undisturbed on plain surface for 20-30 min.
- Eggs depending on their specific gravity and that of the solution float and settle at the surface of the surface.

- Keep a coverslip over the top surface of the tube merely touching the surface and remove.
- Keep the coverslip inverted over a glass slide and examine under microscope at low and high power for the presence of eggs.

2.5.4 Stoll Egg Counting Method (Modified)

This is a simple dilution procedure which facilitates the recognition of eggs and permits a quantitative determination of their concentration in the faeces. Since only 0.01 g of faeces is examined by this method it is not suitable where fewer than 200 eggs are present per gram.

- Place up to 45 glass balls in a shaker jar with 42 ml of water.
- Add 3 g of faeces in the jar and fit the stopper.
- The jar is shaken until all the fecal matter is broken down.
- The mixture is poured through a wire mesh screen with an aperture of 0.15 mm and the strained fluid caught in a bowl. The debris left on the screen is discarded.
- The filtrate of faeces is stirred properly, and 0.15 ml fluid is taken out by means of a graduated pipette.
- The measured quantity of fluid is ejected on to a microscope slide and covered with a 22 x 22 mm cover glass.
- Eggs must be counted in that part of fluid not under the cover glass as well as that beneath the cover glass.
- The total number of eggs present in the 0.15 ml of diluted faeces is multiplied by 100 to give the number of eggs per gram of the original fecal sample.

2.5.5 Modified McMaster Method

This technique provides accurate quantitative results and is widely used in veterinary parasitology.

- Place up to 45 glass balls in a shaker jar and add 42 ml saturated NaCl.
- Add 3 g of faeces in the jar and close the stopper.
- The jar is shaken until all the fecal matter is broken down.
- The mixture is poured through a wire mesh screen with an aperture of 0.15 mm and the strained fluid caught in a bowl. The debris left on the screen is discarded.
- The filtrate of faeces is stirred properly, and 0.15 ml of fluid is taken out by means of a graduated pipette and carefully run into one counting

chamber. After further stirring, a second sample is withdrawn and run into the other chamber.

- All the eggs under the two separate grids are counted. Since 3 g of faeces yielded 45 ml of suspension (1 g per 15 ml suspension) and the volume of suspension examined was 0.3 ml (0.15 ml under each grid of the counting chamber) and the number of eggs per g of faeces is obtained by multiplying the total eggs under the two grids by 50.

2.5.6 Fecal Culture for Coccidia oocyst

Coccidian infections are very common and important for poultry and ruminants especially in young ones. Several species are incriminated for this condition for a specific host species. When passed in faeces the coccidian oocysts are unsporulated and cannot be differentiated. Therefore, culture of fecal samples for sporulation of coccidian oocysts is important for diagnosis as well as epidemiological study.

- Take a small amount (3-5 g) of faeces in a pestle and mortar.
- Add 2.5% potassium dichromate to emulsify it.
- Filter through a strainer.
- Pour the filtrate into petri dish to the depth of ½ cm only.
- Keep at room temperature.
- Examine under microscope at every 6-12 hours for complete sporulation.
- Record shape, size by micrometry and the sporulation time for identification.

2.5.7 Baermann's Technique for Culture of Nematode Parasite Larvae

The method is useful for the isolation of larvae from the faeces, soils, and minced tissue of animals. It is also used for removing and concentrating larvae from coproculture.

Baermann's apparatus consists of a glass funnel of about 10 inches diameter in which is placed a wire gauge of 1 mm mesh and about 9 inches in diameter. On the wire gauge, a muslin cloth is placed. The funnel is joined to a centrifuge tube by means of rubber tube, the latter is provided by a pinch coke. The assembled funnel is placed in a rings stand. The material may be infective and must be handled accordingly.

- Fill the funnel with warm water about 50 °C so that it is as about ½ inches above the layer of cloth with wire gauge. Let the water cool to 40 °C.

- Spread the sample evenly over the cloths and let stand for ½ hour. The larvae will be attracted by the warmth of the water, migrate through the cloth and gauge and collect in the stem of the funnel.

Open the pinch cock and with draw some of the water in a dish for examination. Larvae may be detected with a dissecting microscope and if numerous, some of them removed directly from the dish for identification. If a few or no larvae are seen, a considerable amount of water should be withdrawn and centrifuged and the sediment examined. Largest yield will be obtained by allowing the material to remain in the funnel for 24hours before drawing off the larvae.

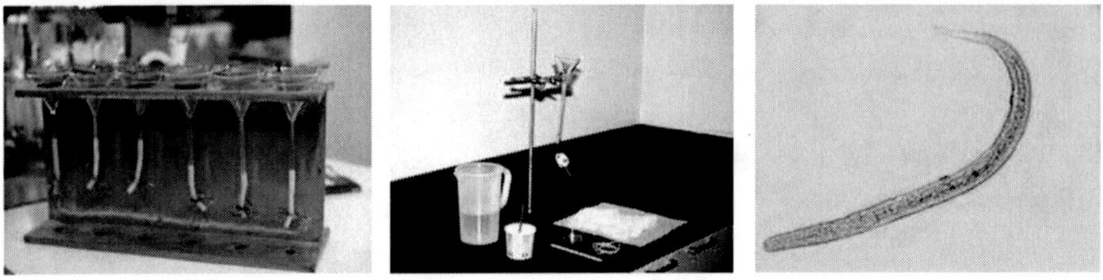

A. Baemann apparatus, B. Baermann technique and C. Nematode larvae(culture)

Fig. 27

2.5.8 Best Practices for Parasitological Examination of Fecal Samples

Sample Collection

- Collect fresh samples directly from the rectum whenever possible
- Gather samples from multiple affected animals in a herd
- Use clean, wide-mouth containers with secure lids
- Label containers with animal ID, date, time, and collection method
- Process samples within 2-3 hours of collection
- Store at 4°C if immediate processing isn't possible

Sample Preparation

- Wear appropriate protective equipment
- Examine samples for consistency, color, and presence of visible parasites
- Use appropriate amounts of sample based on test method:
    - Direct smear: pea-sized amount
    - Floatation: 5-10 grams
    - Sedimentation: 3-5 grams
- Remove foreign material before processing
- Use fresh floatation solutions to ensure proper specific gravity

Examination Techniques

- Start with low magnification (10x) for scanning
- Switch to higher magnification (40x) for detailed observation
- Examine multiple fields per slide
- Focus through different planes while examining
- Document findings with measurements when possible

Interpretation

- Consider animal species, age, and clinical signs
- Account for parasite life cycles when interpreting results
- Evaluate egg/cyst counts in context of clinical presentation
- Consider mixed infections
- Document treatment responses through follow-up examinations

2.6 Serum Biochemistry

Serum biochemistry is an important aid for the diagnosis of infectious and non-infectious diseases conditions. Any damage to cell/tissue/organs cause release of organ specific enzyme and other protein molecules in the plasma. An estimation of the level of these molecules in serum/plasma gives an indication of damage caused. Besides, estimation of various ions sodium, potassium, calcium, phosphorus etc may be used for accessing the health status of the animal.

Requirements

- Serum (Good quality without haemolysis)
- Diagnostic reagent (commercially available) for estimation
- Spectrophotometer

Analysis may be performed immediately after collection or serum may be stored at –20°C for further use.

Methods

As indicated by the manufacturers of the diagnostic reagents (it may vary slightly for different manufacturers)

Clinical Significance

Protein

- Hyperproteinemia is observed in hemoconcentration, dehydration, lactating animals, response to antigen, infectious and suppurative diseases, chronic diseases like tuberculosis, aging etc.

- Relative hypoproteinemia observed in inadequate production in new borne animals, malnutrition, anorexia, inadequate digestion or absorption, chronic hepatopathy, neoplasm of lymphoid tissues and liver, pregnancy. Loss of protein from body in acute blood loss, chronic blood or protein loss in gastrointestinal disorders, parasitism such as immature amphistomosis, haemonchosis, fasciolosis, etc. and renal diseases etc.

Albumin : Hypoalbuminemia seen in

- Malnutrition: Lack of proper amino acids, enzymes and impaired digestion & absorption, diarrhoea
- Liver disease (decrease synthesis) – Cirrhosis, malignancies, necrosis, inflammations
- Increased protein catabolism – fever, infection, trauma, pregnancy
- Nephrotic syndrome - Leakage of albumin through damaged vessels and tissues
- Enteropathy – Increased fecal losses are associated with chronic enteric diseases e.g. Johne's disease, enteritis, ulcerative colitis, parasitism, abomasal disorders, intestinal neoplasm etc.

Alkaline Phosphatase: Serum alkaline phosphatase is increased in disease of bone including metastasis, rickets and healing fractures. Elevations are seen in growing animals.

Blood Glucose: Glucose estimations provide valuable information about the course, severity and therapeutic control of diabetes mellitus.

Urea: Low values indicate protein malnutrition and liver damage. Increased value indicates the serious impairment of renal function. In the chronic renal failure, urea correlates better with the symptom of uremia.

Creatinine: Serum creatinine is more specific and sensitive indicator of renal function than serum urea. Low values have no significance. The increased values indicate renal impairment, generalised renal disease and reduced glomerular filtration rate.

Uric Acid : Increase in serum uric acid concentrations are seen in liver damage, gout - in which salts of uric acid are deposited in and around joints. Increased uric acid levels are also seen in polycythemia, leukemia, pernnicious anemia, chronic hemolytic anemia, lymphosarcoma and treatment with cytotoxic drugs.

Table 6: Normal values of serum biochemistry (g/dl) in different animals

Species	Dog	Cat	Horse	Cattle	Sheep	Goat	Pig	Man	Mithun
Total Protein (g/dl)	5–7	6–7.5	6–8	5.5–7	5–7.5	5–7.5	5.5–7.5	6–8	6–8
Albumin (g/dl)	3–4	2.7 – 3.2	2.8 – 3.0	2.7 – 3.9	3.0	3.95	1.9 – 3.4	4 – 5	3–4
SGPT/APT (IU/L)	5–24	2 – 14	1–6	4–11	10–12	7–24	9–17	up to 40	20–35
SGOT/ AST(IU/L)	6–13	6–11	58–94	20–34	70–90	43–132	8–22	up to 35	85–120
Alkaline Phosphatase (IU/L)	3–16	2–7	11–31	0–38	5–30	7–30	9–31	20 – 150	20–120
Glucose (mg/dl)	70–110	70–110	75–115	45–75	50–80	50–75	85–150	65–120	60–120
Creatinine (mg/dl)	1.0 – 2.0	1.0 – 2.0	1.0 – 2.0	1.0 – 2.0	1.0 – 2.0	1.0 – 2.0	1.0 – 2.0	0.8 – 1.4	1.0–2.0
Urea (mg/dl)	10–30	10–30	10–30	10–30	10–30	10–30	10–30	15–40	15–25
Cholesterol (mg/dl)	125 –250	95 – 130	75 – 150	80 – 120	50 – 75	80 – 130	35 – 55	100 –150	90–120
Uric acid (mg/dl)	3.0 –7.5	3.0 – 7.5	3.0 – 7.5	3.0 – 7.5	3.0 – 7.5	3.0 – 7.5	3.0 – 7.5	2.6–7.2	2.5–7.0

2.7 Immunodiagnostic Assays

Introduction

Immunodiagnostic methods are used extensively for diagnosis of diseases. These tests detect and measure specific molecules by exploiting the precise binding between antibodies and their target antigens. Most commonly used methods are those using labeled antigen and antibody.

1 Immunoperoxidase test
2. Immunofluorescence test and
3. Enzyme Linked Immunosorbent Assay (ELISA)

Immunoperoxidase tests are commonly used for identifying antigens in tissue sections while immunofluorescence and ELISA are generally used for serum and other biological fluid samples. Immunofluorescence is an antigen-antibody reaction where the antibodies are tagged (labelled) with a fluorescent dye and the antigen-antibody complex is visualised using ultra-violet (fluorescent) microscope. Fluorochromes are dyes that absorb ultra-violet rays and emit visible light through a process called fluorescence. Immunofluorescence is used for identification of infectious agents in clinical samples. Fluorescent antibody methods are time consuming and require expensive UV microscope.

2.7.1 Enzyme Linked Immunosorbent Assay (ELISA)

Enzyme linked immunosorbent assay (ELISA) is a non-radioactive immunoassay in which the antigen and antibody complex is detected by using specific enzyme labeled antibody conjugate and substrate. It is simple, sensitive, specific and precise and is the most commonly used diagnostic method for serological diagnosis of a number of diseases caused by various pathogens.

Principle

The ELISA technique detects antigen-antibody complexes through color reactions using enzymes and their specific substrates. Either antigens or antibodies can be attached to a solid surface (usually a plastic plate).

For antigen detection: The unknown antigen binds to capture antibodies on the plate. Then, enzyme-linked detection antibodies are added that specifically bind to the antigen. If the antigen is present, a complex forms and stays bound to the plate.

For antibody detection: Known antigens are coated on the plate. Sample containing unknown antibodies is added, followed by enzyme-linked secondary antibodies that bind to the unknown antibodies.

In both cases, adding the appropriate substrate causes the enzyme to produce a color change. This color can be observed by eye or measured more precisely using an ELISA reader (spectrophotometer). There are different types of ELISA test such as:

- Direct ELISA
- Indirect ELISA
- Sandwich ELISA/Immunocapture ELISA
- Competitive ELISA
- Liquid phase blocking sandwich ELISA
- Liquid phase blocking competition ELISA

Materials Required

Plastic wares: e.g. Solid phase (96 well ELISA microplates), single and multichannel pipettes, microtips etc.

Washing buffers: Usually PBS or Tris -buffered saline (pH 7.4) with detergent such as 0.05% (v/v) Tween20 (TBST).

Coating buffer: Antigen or antibodies should be diluted in coating buffer to immobilise them to the wells. Carbonate/bicarbonate buffer (100mM, pH 9.6) or PBS (pH 7.4) is used to coat the plate with second antibody to enhance the sensitivity of the assay. Bicarbonate/carbonate coating buffer (100 mM) consists of Na2CO_3 (3.03 g), $NaHCO_3$ (6.0 g) and distilled water (1000 ml).

Blocking buffer: Any one of few immunologically inert substances e.g. Bovine serum albumin fraction V (1% BSA), Fetal calf serum (FCS) (1-5%), horse serum (1-5%), lactalbumin hydrolysate (1-5%) and skimmed milk powder (3-5%), casein or gelatin can be used in PBS as blocking buffer. Primary and secondary antibody should be diluted in 1x blocking solution to prevent adsorption of nonspecific protein to the ELISA pate wells.

Enzymes: Horseradish peroxidase (HRP), alkaline phosphatase, β galactosidase, glucose oxidase and urease, HRP is the enzyme of choice because it gives satisfactory and reproducible results and is available commercially.

Substrate solution: Substrate to be used is specific for the type of enzymes as follows:

Enzyme	**Substrate**
Horse Radish Peroxidase	Ortho-phenylene diamine (OPD) and H_2O_2
Alkaline phosphatase	p-nitrophenyl phosphate
β galactosidase	O-nitrophenyl-D-galactoside (ONDG)

Prepare fresh OPD solution (4.0 mg of OPD powder in 10.0 ml of 0.1 M sodium citrate buffer, pH 5.0) just before use. Add H_2O_2 (1µl/ml) to the OPD solution immediately before use in the test.

Stopping reagent: 1(M) H_2SO_4 (54 ml H_2SO_4 in 946 ml DW)

Safety Note: Always add acid to the water not vice versa and store at RT.

Direct ELISA

This assay can be used to detect unknown antigen or antibody. If antigen is unknown, then known specific antibody and if antibody is unknown then a known antigen should be used for labeling with enzyme.

General Procedure

Coating antigen to microplate

- Dilute the antigen to a final concentration of 20µg/ml in PBS or other carbonate buffer. Coat the wells of ELISA plate with the antigen by pipetting 50 µl of the diluted antigen in the top wells of the plate. Dilute down the plate as required. Antigen concentration (20µg/ml) will saturate most of the binding sites in the wells.

- Cover the plate with an adhesive plastic and incubate for 2 h at room temperature, or 4°C overnight. The coating incubation time may require some optimisation.
- Remove the coating solution and wash the plate twice by filling the wells with 200 μl PBS. The solutions or washes are removed by flicking the plate over a sink. The remaining drops are removed by patting the plate on a paper towel.

Blocking

- Block the remaining protein-binding sites in the coated wells by adding 200 μl blocking buffer, 5% non-fat dry milk/PBS, per well. Alternative blocking reagents include BlockACE or BSA.
- Cover the plate with an adhesive plastic and incubate for at least 2 h at room temperature or, if more convenient, overnight at 4°C.
- Wash the plate twice with PBS.

Incubation with the Antibody

- Add 100 μl of the antibody, diluted at the optimal concentration (according to the manufacturer's instructions) in blocking buffer immediately before use.
- Cover the plate with an adhesive plastic and incubate for 2 h at room temperature. This incubation time may require optimisation. Although 2 hours is usually enough to obtain a strong signal, if a weak signal is obtained, stronger staining will often be observed when incubated overnight at 4°C.
- Wash the plate four times with PBS.

Detection

- Dispense 100 μl (or 50 μl) of the substrate solution per well with a multichannel pipette.
- After sufficient color development (if it is necessary) add 100 μl of stop solution to the wells.
- Read the absorbance (optical density) of each well with a plate reader.

Safety Note: some enzyme substrates are considered hazardous (potential carcinogens), therefore always handle with care and wear gloves.

Analysis of data: Prepare a standard curve from the data produced from the serial dilutions with concentration on the x axis (log scale) vs absorbance on the Y axis (linear). Interpolate the concentration of the sample from this standard curve.

Interpretation: Color development indicates positive reaction. Intensity of the color is proportionate to the amount of antigen or antibody complex on the solid phase.

Advantage: Very simple and less time-consuming.

Disadvantage: Nonspecific reaction if crude antigen is used for coating. There is a need to procure/prepare conjugate against all the pathogens.

Indirect ELISA

Indirect ELISA detects antibodies in a sample by using an antigen-coated plate, followed by a secondary antibody conjugated to an enzyme for signal amplification.

Procedure

- Coat the ELISA plate with purified known antigen diluted in coating buffer and incubate at 4°C overnight or at 37°C for 1 hour.
- Wash with washing buffer for at least 3 times.
- Add serum samples/antibody in blocking buffer and incubate at 37°C for 1 hour.
- Wash with washing buffer for at least 3 times.
- Add enzyme labeled anti-species antibody (conjugate) in blocking buffer and incubate at 37°C for 1 hour.
- Wash with washing buffer for at least 3 times.
- Add substrate solution and keep the plate in the dark for 10-15 min. Stop the reaction by adding stopping reagent and look for color development visually or read in ELISA reader.

Advantage: More specific for detection and quantification of unknown antibody in serum samples.

Disadvantage: More time consuming and require anti species antibody.

Anti species antibody is prepared against the normal globulin of species from which serum samples are tested. For example, if the serum samples are tested from sheep then anti-sheep antibody is prepared in other species like rabbit by using normal ovine globulin.

Sandwich ELISA

This assay is also called capture or trapping assay, because it is used to capture or trap antigen by specific antibody passively adsorbed on the solid phase.

Certain antigen cannot be used to coat ELISA pates directly because of their very low concentration or due to the presence of high concentration of contaminating protein or any other unknown antigen from crude mixture. Such antigen can be detected by this assay.

- Coat ELISA plate with specific antibody (example, rabbit antibody against goat pox virus) solution diluted in coating buffer and incubate at 4°C overnight or at 37°C for 1 hour.
- Wash the plate with washing buffer for at least 3 times.
- Add antigen (goat pox virus) solution diluted in blocking buffer and incubate at 37°C for 1 hour.
- Wash the plate with washing buffer for at least 3 times.
- Add antibody (guinea pig antibody against goat pox virus) directed against antigen. Incubate at 37°C for 1 hour.
- Wash the plate with washing buffer for at least 3 times.
- Add conjugate (anti-guinea pig globulin coupled with enzyme) and incubate at 37°C for 1 hour.
- Wash the plate with washing buffer for at least 3 times.
- Add substrate solution and keep the plate in the dark for 10-15 min. Stop the reaction with stopping reagent and read and look for color development. Read the result in ELISA reader.

Advantage: Specific for detection of unknown antigen present in very low level or in crude mixture.

Disadvantage: Antibodies against the antigen raised in two species are required.

Competitive ELISA

Used to identify and quantify unknown antibody and to compare the relative affinity of binding of antibodies for the same antigen.

- Coat the ELISA plate with purified antigen after diluting in coating buffer. Incubate at 4°C overnight or at 37°C for 1 hour.
- Wash the plate with washing buffer for at least 3 times.
- Add the test serum sample against the antigen, followed by addition of the monoclonal antibody directed against the same antigen and incubate at 37°C for 1 hour.
- Wash the plate with washing buffer for at least 3 times.
- Add enzyme-labeled secondary antibody specific to the monoclonal antibody species (conjugate) and incubate at 37°C for 1 hour.
- Wash the plate with washing buffer for at least 3 times.
- Add substrate solution and keep for 10-15 minutes in dark and stop the reaction and read the results.

Interpretation

- No color development indicates the specificity of the test antibody and complete saturation of binding sites of the antigen by the test antibody leaving no binding site for the secondary antibody (monoclonal) and then to labeled antibody.
- Less color indicates low concentration of the test antibody leaving some binding sites for the secondary antibody (monoclonal) and then to labeled antibody.
- Intense color development indicates that the suspected test antibody is not specific for the antigen leaving all binding sites for the secondary antibody (monoclonal) and then to labeled antibody.

SUMMARY

Direct ELISA (for detection of antigen)

Test antigen + Antibody against that particular antigen coupled with enzyme (conjugate) + substrate = Color or no color.

Color: positive for that particular antigen.

No color: Negative for that particular antigen.

Indirect ELISA (for detection of antibody)

Known antigen + test antibody + anti-species antibody coupled with enzyme (conjugate) + substrate = Color or no color.

Color: positive for that particular antibody.

No color: Negative for that particular antibody.

Sandwich ELISA (for detection of antigen)

Antibody against the known antigen + test antigen + Antibody against the known antigen in different spaces + Anti-species antibodies coupled with enzyme (conjugate) + substrate = Color or no color.

Color: Positive for that particular antigen.

No color: Negative for that particular antigen.

Competitive ELISA (for detection of antibody)

Known antigen + test antibody & monoclonal antibody against the antigen + anti-mouse immunoglobulin coupled with enzyme (conjugate) + substrate = Color or no color.

Color: Negative for the particular antibody.

No color: Positive for the particular antibody.

Please refer to Appendix B6 for issues and troubleshooting related to ELISA

2.7.2 Using an ELISA washer and reader

1. ELISA washer

- Program the washer to dispense the washing buffer gently into wells without dislodging the coated antigen or bound antibodies.
- Perform 3-5 washes for each step, ensuring complete removal of previous reagents.
- Check for uniformity and dryness of wells after washing.

2. ELISA reader

- Calibrate the reader according to the manufacturer's instructions.
- Use a blank well (no antigen) to zero the reader.
- Insert the plate into the reader, ensuring correct alignment.
- Set the wavelength according to the substrate used (e.g., 450 nm for TMB).
- Record absorbance values and analyse results accordingly.

2.7.3 Best practices and techniques for ELISA

Sample preparation

- Use freshly prepared or properly stored samples to prevent degradation.
- Avoid repeated freeze-thaw cycles to preserve sample integrity.
- Dilute samples appropriately to fall within the assay's detection range.

Plate coating

- Use high-quality, antigen-specific capture antibodies for coating plates in sandwich ELISA.
- Optimise coating conditions (antibody concentration, pH, and incubation time) for uniform binding.
- Block nonspecific binding sites with an effective blocking buffer (e.g., BSA, casein, or gelatin).

Antibody selection

- Use highly specific primary antibodies to reduce cross-reactivity.
- Choose enzyme-conjugated secondary antibodies that are specific to the primary antibody species.

Reagent handling

- Prepare fresh reagents and dilutions on the day of the experiment.

- Ensure all reagents are at room temperature before use unless otherwise specified.
- Use consistent pipetting techniques to avoid variability.

Washing steps

- Wash plates thoroughly after each step to reduce background noise.
- Use an automated plate washer if available for uniform washing.
- Ensure no residual liquid remains in wells after washing.

Incubation conditions

- Maintain uniform temperature and time for all wells during incubations.
- Use a plate shaker if the protocol recommends it to enhance binding efficiency.

Substrate handling

- Prepare substrate solution just before use, as some substrates are light- or time-sensitive.
- Protect light-sensitive substrates (e.g., TMB) from exposure to light.
- Stop the reaction at the same time for all wells to maintain consistency.

Controls and standards

- Include positive and negative controls for quality assurance.
- Use a standard curve with known concentrations for quantification.

Data accuracy

- Perform all samples and standards in duplicate or triplicate to reduce variability.
- Monitor plate edge effects; avoid using edge wells if they tend to show variation.

Storage and handling

- Store plates, antibodies, and reagents at recommended conditions to preserve activity.
- Use aseptic techniques to prevent contamination of reagents or samples.

Equipment calibration

- Regularly calibrate plate readers, pipettes, and other equipment.
- Ensure uniform pipetting to avoid volume inconsistencies between wells.

By following these best practices, you can maximize ELISA sensitivity, specificity, and reproducibility.

3

Essential Techniques in Molecular Biology

This chapter outlines fundamental molecular biology protocols essential for genomic analysis and molecular characterisation. Modern molecular biology relies heavily on precise analytical techniques for studying genetic material. Hence, this section presents a typical workflow encompassing nucleic acid extraction, amplification, and subsequent analysis. These methodologies are fundamental to various applications in molecular biology, including phylogenetic analysis, gene expression studies, and molecular diagnostics.

The chapter covers four core molecular biology and bioinformatics techniques, each building upon the previous:

1. Genomic DNA Extraction: Protocols for efficient isolation of DNA from biological samples. This encompasses cell lysis, protein denaturation, and nucleic acid purification through standard separation techniques. The quality and purity of extracted DNA significantly influences downstream applications.
2. Primer Design with Primer3: In silico design of oligonucleotide primers for PCR amplification. This section covers primer design parameters including optimal melting temperature (Tm), GC content, primer length, and considerations for avoiding secondary structures and primer-dimer formation.
3. Polymerase Chain Reaction (PCR) Amplification and Gel Electrophoresis: Detailed protocols for PCR optimisation and amplicon analysis. This includes:
   a) Components necessary for PCR
   b) Thermal cycling parameters
   c) Standard procedure for PCR
   d) Agarose gel electrophoresis for amplicon visualisation and size determination

4. Sequence Alignment using MAFFT: Implementation of multiple sequence alignment (MSA) algorithms for comparative genomic analysis. This section covers:
    a) Key factors to consider for multiple sequence alignment (MSA).
    b) Steps to perform MSA with MAFFT.
    c) Applications of MSA

These techniques form an integrated workflow essential for molecular characterisation

1. Initial DNA extraction provides template material for downstream analysis
2. PCR amplification, guided by rationally designed primers, enables selective amplification of target sequences
3. Gel electrophoresis confirms successful amplification and provides preliminary size analysis
4. Sequence alignment facilitates comparative analysis of amplified regions

These methodologies are fundamental to various applications in molecular biology, including:

- Molecular phylogenetics
- Population genetics
- Molecular diagnostics
- Genetic variation analysis
- Evolutionary studies

The protocols outlined here represent standard operating procedures followed in veterinary parasitology laboratories initiating molecular work from collected field or clinical specimens. Familiarity with these techniques—and understanding how they connect within an experimental pipeline—is essential for effectively designing and troubleshooting molecular assays. Mastery of these foundational methods provides the basis for more advanced analyses such as species genotyping, detection of resistance alleles, or comparative genomics in parasitic organisms.

3.1 Genomic DNA Extraction

3.1.1 Principle of DNA Extraction

DNA Extraction is a fundamental laboratory technique that involves isolating genomic DNA from biological samples, such as blood, tissues, or cells, in a controlled environment. At its core, DNA extraction is based on disrupting cellular membranes and protein complexes to release the DNA while removing contaminants, such as proteins, lipids, and carbohydrates. The extracted DNA can then be used for various downstream applications, including PCR, sequencing, genotyping, and genetic analysis. By carefully selecting and applying extraction techniques, researchers can obtain high-quality genetic material suitable for precise molecular investigations.

Why is DNA Extraction Important?

DNA extraction is a key process in numerous scientific and medical fields, serving as a fundamental technique with far-reaching implications. It provides researchers and medical professionals with access to an organism's genetic blueprint, enabling critical investigations across multiple domains. In medical diagnostics, DNA extraction allows for genetic testing, disease identification, and personalised medicine approaches. In forensic science, it helps solve criminal investigations by analysing trace genetic evidence. In veterinary science, DNA extraction plays a vital role in diagnosing genetic diseases, studying animal populations, and understanding genetic diversity in different species. Researchers use DNA extraction to study genetic variations, understand evolutionary relationships, conduct genetic engineering, and explore genomic characteristics of various organisms. From identifying genetic disorders to tracking infectious diseases, from archaeological genetics to conservation biology, DNA extraction is the key that unlocks genetic information, providing knowledge that were once impossible to obtain.

3.1.2 Types of Biological Samples

Biological samples for DNA extraction encompass a wide range of source materials, each presenting unique challenges and requirements for successful genetic material isolation. Common sources include:

Blood: Blood is particularly valuable for DNA extraction because white blood cells (leukocytes) contain nuclei, unlike red blood cells which lose their nuclei during maturation. A single millilitre of human blood contains approximately 4,000-11,000 leukocytes, making it an extremely rich source of genomic DNA. The presence of anticoagulants like EDTA or heparin in collected samples prevents clotting and helps maintain DNA integrity.

Tissue Samples: Tissue samples present varying challenges depending on their state. Fresh tissues offer the highest quality DNA but require immediate processing or proper preservation to prevent nuclease activity. Frozen tissues (typically stored at -80°C) maintain DNA integrity well but can form ice crystals that disrupt cellular structures. Formalin-fixed, paraffin-embedded

(FFPE) tissues, common in clinical settings, often yield fragmented DNA due to crosslinking between proteins and nucleic acids.

Cultured Cells: Cultured cells provide a controlled environment for DNA extraction. Laboratory-grown mammalian, bacterial or other cells eliminate many variables present in clinical samples, making them ideal for standardised protocols. However, contamination with mycoplasma or other microorganisms can introduce foreign DNA, which necessitates regular testing and validation of cell line purity.

Saliva: Saliva is increasingly popular for genetic testing due to its non-invasive collection. The oral epithelial cells shed naturally into saliva contain nuclear DNA, though the quality can be affected by bacterial contamination and nuclease activity. Stabilising solutions are often used to preserve DNA integrity during collection and transport.

Hair Roots: Hair roots, specifically the follicular tags attached to plucked hairs, contain cellular material rich in nuclear DNA. The keratin-based hair shaft itself contains minimal nuclear DNA but can provide mitochondrial DNA. This source is particularly useful in wildlife studies where non-invasive sampling is crucial.

Forensic Samples: Forensic samples represent perhaps the most challenging category. These samples often contain degraded DNA due to environmental exposure and are frequently present in minute quantities.

It is important to remember that each source material requires specific optimisation of extraction protocols, and the following factors should be considered:

- Cell membrane composition and the appropriate lysis conditions
- Presence of inhibitors that might affect downstream applications
- Storage requirements to maintain sample integrity
- The expected DNA yield and quality needed for specific applications

3.1.3 DNA Extraction Methods

In order to successfully isolate high quality DNA, it is important to carefully select and optimise the extraction protocols. These methods must effectively balance the need to separate the DNA from cellular structures while preventing degradation and maintaining purity. The choice of protocol depends heavily on the source material, downstream applications, and required DNA quality. Modern extraction techniques combine traditional chemical and mechanical approaches with advanced purification technologies, thus offering researchers a complete toolkit for handling diverse biological samples. The different methods that are generally used for DNA extraction is briefly discussed below.

Chemical Lysis Methods

Cell lysis is the critical first step in DNA extraction, where cellular and nuclear membranes are broken down to release genetic material. This typically involves a multi-component lysis buffer containing detergents such as SDS (Sodium Dodecyl Sulfate) or Triton X-100 that solubilise lipid membranes by interfering with lipid-lipid and lipid-protein interactions. Chaotropic salts (guanidinium thiocyanate or guanidinium chloride) then denature proteins and inactivate nucleases. Proteinase K, a broad-spectrum serine protease digests proteins that might be bound to DNA, including histones from chromatin structures that can interfere with downstream applications. Buffer components (usually Tris-HCl) maintain optimal pH for enzymatic activity.

The effectiveness of chemical lysis varies significantly with sample type. For instance, gram-positive bacteria require stronger lysis conditions due to their peptidoglycan cell wall, often necessitating additional enzymes such as lysozyme.

Mechanical Disruption Techniques

In some cases, chemical lysis alone is insufficient and mechanical disruption techniques become essential when dealing with samples that resist chemical lysis alone, such as tough plant tissues, fungi, or gram-positive bacteria with rigid cell walls. Bead beating involves agitating samples with ceramic, glass, or metal beads of specific sizes chosen based on the sample type and desired fragmentation level. Sonication uses ultrasonic waves to create cavitation bubbles that, upon collapse, generate enough force to shear cellular components. Homogenisation through grinding with liquid nitrogen freezes samples brittle enough to be pulverised effectively while preventing thermal degradation of DNA. The challenge lies in finding the right balance between sufficient disruption and avoiding excessive DNA shearing, which could compromise downstream applications.

Each method has specific applications. For example, bead beating is particularly effective for yeast and plant tissues, while sonication works well for bacterial cells but can fragment DNA if overused.

Silica-based and Magnetic Bead Extraction

Silica-based and magnetic bead extraction methods have revolutionised DNA purification by offering highly efficient and automatable processes. Silica-based methods exploit DNA's ability to bind to silica surfaces under high-chaotropic salt conditions and low pH, while proteins and other cellular components remain unbound. The bound DNA can then be washed with ethanol-containing buffers to remove impurities before elution in low-salt conditions. Magnetic bead technology uses particles with a magnetite core coated with silica or carboxyl groups that bind DNA under specific buffer conditions. These beads can be easily manipulated with magnetic fields, allowing for efficient separation and washing steps. The choice between these methods often depends on sample throughput requirements and the presence of potential inhibitors.

3.1.4 DNA Extraction using Spin-Column Based Kits

In this manual, we will focus on spin column-based DNA extraction, a modern technique that leverages silica membrane technology to efficiently bind, wash, and elute DNA. Spin columns provide a quick, clean method for isolating high-quality genomic DNA, with the ability to process multiple samples simultaneously. This technique offers several advantages, including reduced hands-on time, minimal use of hazardous chemicals, and reproducible results across different biological sample types.

Spin column-based DNA extraction involves the following steps:

- *Cell Lysis:* The first step involves lysing the cells to release genomic DNA. Lysis buffer, containing detergents and chaotropic salts, disrupts cell membranes, nuclear envelopes, and protein complexes, facilitating the release of DNA into the solution.
- *Binding to Spin Column:* The lysate is then transferred to a spin column containing a silica membrane. Silica has a high affinity for DNA, allowing the DNA molecules to selectively bind to the membrane while contaminants, such as proteins and polysaccharides, are removed through the wash steps.
- *Washing Steps:* Wash buffers are used to remove impurities and cellular debris that may interfere with downstream applications. These buffers contain ethanol, which helps to wash away contaminants while allowing DNA to remain bound to the silica membrane.
- *DNA Elution:* Elution buffer is added directly to the spin column, disrupting the interactions between DNA and the silica membrane. This releases the purified DNA into the eluate, which is collected by centrifugation into a clean microcentrifuge tube. Elution buffer typically contains a low ionic strength solution, such as TE buffer or water, to promote DNA recovery.
- *Quality Control:* The extracted DNA is then assessed for quantity, purity, and integrity using spectrophotometric analysis and agarose gel electrophoresis. Spectrophotometric analysis measures DNA concentration based on its absorbance at specific wavelengths, while gel electrophoresis evaluates DNA size and purity based on its migration pattern through an agarose gel.

- *Documentation and Storage:* The results of the quality control analysis are documented, and the extracted DNA is properly labelled and stored at appropriate temperatures (-20°C or -80°C) for future use in downstream molecular biology applications.

Standard Protocol for DNA extraction using spin column-based kits

Important: Specific buffer (lysis, wash, elution) composition may vary depending on manufacturer and kit. Preparation of these buffers must be done according to kit instruction.

Sample preparation

Tissue

Cut tissue into small pieces and place in a 1.5 ml microcentrifuge tube with lysis buffer (typically 10–20 µl buffer per mg tissue). Add Proteinase K at a final concentration of **100–200 µg/ml of homogenate** (e.g., 1 µl of 20 mg/ml stock per 100–200 µl buffer). Mix by vortexing and incubate at 56°C *(some protocols require 37°C)* until completely lysed, vortexing occasionally. Briefly vortex for 15 seconds before proceeding to DNA extraction.

Blood

Add Proteinase K to a final concentration of **100–200 µg/ml** in the lysate. Mix anticoagulated blood (typically 5–10 µl) with Phosphate-Buffered Saline (PBS) to reach a total volume of ~200–220 µl. Vortex and incubate at 56°C until lysed.

Cultured cells

Pellet up to **5 × 10^6 cells** by centrifugation (5 min, 300 × g), resuspend in 200 µl PBS, and add Proteinase K (final 100–200 µg/ml). Vortex and incubate at 56°C until lysed.

Notes:

- *Complete lysis depends on sample type. Tissue digestion may require longer incubation times, sometimes overnight.*
- *Some protocols recommend additional reagents apart from PBS to enhance lysis.*

1. Add ethanol (96–100%) at a **1:1 ratio** to the lysate volume. Mix thoroughly by vortexing to ensure proper DNA binding to the matrix.
2. Pipette the mixture into a spin column placed in a collection tube. Centrifuge at ≥6000 x g (8000 rpm) for ~1 minute to collect the DNA on the column. Discard the flow-through and collection tube.

3. Place the spin column in a new collection tube. Add **2–2.5 volumes of wash buffer 1** (relative to original lysate volume). Centrifuge for ~1 minute at ≥6000 x g to wash the DNA-bound matrix. Discard the flow-through and collection tube.
4. Place the spin column in a new collection tube. Add **2–2.5 volumes of wash buffer 2** (relative to original lysate volume) to the column. Centrifuge for ~3 minutes at 20,000 x g (14,000 rpm) to remove residual contaminants. Discard the flow-through and collection tube.
5. Transfer the spin column to a new microcentrifuge tube to collect the purified DNA.
6. Elute the DNA by adding **elution buffer (typically 0.5–1× the original lysate volume)** to the center of the spin column membrane. Incubate for ~1 minute at room temperature (15–25°C) to allow the DNA to dissolve. (*Depending on the kit, warming the elution buffer to 60-70°C can increase elution efficiency and increase DNA yield).*
7. Centrifuge for ~1 minute at ≥6000 x g to collect the eluted DNA. *(Repeat this step for increased DNA yield)*

   Please refer to Appendix C1 for common issues and troubleshooting.

3.1.5 Best Practice and Techniques for DNA Extraction

- EDTA is the preferred anticoagulant for blood samples, as it can be easily removed during purification and does not interfere with DNA yield and purity. Sodium citrate is the second-best choice, while heparin should be avoided due to its negative impact on DNA yield and downstream PCR analyses.
- To preserve DNA integrity in samples, minimise exposure to sunlight and temperatures above 4°C, as UV radiation and heat can degrade DNA. Stabilizing reagents (e.g., Tris-EDTA buffer) or specialized DNA preservative solutions can also be added to further inhibit degradation.
- Refrigerating or freezing samples quickly is crucial. Refrigerate samples at 4°C if they'll be used within three days, as rapid refrigeration enhances DNA yield. Conversely, freeze samples at -80°C if processing is delayed beyond three days, ideally within two hours of collection to avoid yield reduction.
- Avoid haemolysis (lysing red blood cells) by handling your sample gently. Mix sample only if necessary by gentle inversion. Besides gentle handling, some anticoagulants contribute to haemolysis (e.g., excess EDTA can cause RBC shrinkage). If using EDTA, maintain the correct

volume-to-blood ratio— typically 1.5–2 mg of K_2EDTA per mL of blood — to minimize unwanted effects.

- To maintain enzyme integrity, avoid excessive freeze-thaw cycles by using aliquots of enzyme-containing buffers. Enzymes like Proteinase K and polymerases are particularly sensitive to freeze-thaw cycles. Some labs store aliquots at -20°C in glycerol to improve enzyme stability over multiple uses. If procedures fail, consider using fresh enzyme aliquots.
- When handling DNA pellets post-extraction, take care not to over-dry them during alcohol precipitation. If resuspending difficulties arise, heat the DNA pellet with the rehydration buffer at 5555°C for approximately 5 minutes to facilitate dissolution. Beyond heating at 55°C, using low-ionic-strength buffers (e.g., 0.1X TE) or adding gentle agitation can improve resuspension efficiency.

3.1.6 Importance of DNA Quality and Purity

DNA quality assessment is a critical checkpoint since the reliability of downstream applications depends heavily on both the quantity and integrity of isolated genetic material. While no single method provides complete characterisation, a combination of analytical techniques allows researchers to evaluate different aspects of DNA quality, concentration, purity, and structural integrity. The choice of quality assessment methods depends on the intended downstream application and the nature of the sample material.

Spectrophotometric analysis: This technique utilises UV absorbance at 260nm to determine DNA concentration, while the A260/A280 ratio (optimally ~1.8) indicates protein contamination levels. The A260/A230 ratio (~2.0-2.2) shows organic contaminant presence. However, this method has limitations in that it cannot distinguish between DNA and RNA and cannot determine DNA integrity or fragmentation states.

Gel electrophoresis: a visual assessment tool for DNA integrity and fragmentation patterns, this technique can identify RNA contamination, distinguish between genomic and plasmid DNA, and provide size distribution information for DNA fragments. Although relatively simple, it can provide an idea about sample quality and can help estimate concentration when run against known standards. Capillary electrophoresis is a similar technique but provides greater resolution and specificity by using thin capillaries for separating samples based on size, charge, or other properties.

Fluorometric quantification: DNA-specific dyes such as PicoGreen or SYBR Green provide more accurate measurements, particularly for low DNA concentrations, and can differentiate between double-stranded and single-stranded DNA.

Real-time PCR (qPCR): provides absolute quantification of amplifiable DNA and is particularly valuable for species-specific quantification and evaluation of degraded or mixed samples.

Digital PCR: a powerful tool for absolute quantification without the need for standard curves. This method is excellent for low copy number samples as well as complex or degraded samples.

3.1.7 Applications of DNA extraction

1. **Genetic research:** DNA extraction is foundational in studying gene structure, function, and regulation. It enables the analysis of specific genes or entire genomes, facilitating advancements in understanding hereditary traits, gene expression, and evolutionary biology. Techniques like PCR, sequencing, and cloning rely on high-quality DNA extraction to investigate genetic variations, mutations, and relationships among species.
2. **Medicine and diagnostics:** In clinical settings, DNA extraction supports the detection and diagnosis of genetic disorders such as cystic fibrosis, sickle cell anemia, and cancer. It is crucial for identifying pathogenic microorganisms in infectious diseases and for guiding personalised medicine by analysing a patient's genetic makeup to tailor treatment plans.
3. **Veterinary science:** In veterinary medicine, DNA extraction is applied to diagnose diseases in animals, study genetic markers for breeding programs, and monitor zoonotic pathogens that can transfer between animals and humans. For instance, it aids in identifying parasites, bacteria, and viruses affecting livestock like mithun or domestic ruminants, ensuring better disease management and improved animal welfare. It is also instrumental in wildlife conservation efforts, such as genetic monitoring of endangered species.
4. **Agriculture and food science:** DNA extraction is essential for improving agricultural productivity and sustainability. It supports genetic engineering to develop crops with desirable traits, such as drought resistance, pest tolerance, or higher nutritional value. Marker-assisted breeding programs for livestock rely on DNA extraction to identify genetic markers associated with specific traits. It also plays a role in food safety, enabling the detection of contaminants, allergens, and genetically modified organisms in food products.
5. **Forensic science:** Forensics heavily depends on DNA extraction for identifying individuals in criminal investigations, paternity tests,

and missing persons cases. Extracted DNA from hair, blood, or other biological materials allows the creation of genetic profiles used to match evidence with suspects or victims. Advances in this field have also improved the accuracy of disaster victim identification and historical analyses.

6. **Environmental science:** In ecological and environmental studies, DNA extraction is used to assess biodiversity, monitor microbial communities, and study ecosystem health. Environmental DNA (eDNA) extracted from soil, water, or air samples helps detect invasive species, track endangered wildlife, and understand ecological interactions without directly disturbing the environment.
7. **Biotechnology and industry:** Biotechnological applications of DNA extraction include the development of genetically modified organisms for research, agriculture, and pharmaceuticals. It is critical in creating recombinant DNA technologies for producing vaccines, therapeutic proteins, and other industrial bioproducts. DNA extraction also supports synthetic biology by providing a foundation for designing and engineering new biological systems.

These broad applications show the importance of DNA extraction in advancing knowledge and solving practical problems across multiple disciplines.

3.2 Designing Oligonucleotide Primers for PCR Amplification

Primer design is a fundamental aspect of molecular biology that plays a critical role in Polymerase Chain Reaction (PCR) success. Primers are short DNA sequences, also known as oligonucleotides, that bind specifically to a target DNA region and guide DNA polymerase to amplify the desired segment. Properly designed primers ensure the specificity and efficiency of PCR, minimising unintended products and optimising the amplification process. This section will explore what primer design entails, considerations for designing primers and how to use software such as Primer3 for efficient primer design.

What is Primer Design?

In PCR, primers serve as starting points for DNA synthesis, helping DNA polymerase initiate replication precisely at the target region. Designing these primers involves selecting DNA sequences that:

1. **Have optimal length** for specificity and proper annealing to template.
2. **Have optimal melting temperatures** (Tm) for stable binding without unintended annealing.

3. **Produce optimal amplicon size** that is on the range of 300-1000 base pairs (bp) for standard PCR and 50-150 bp for real-time PCR.
4. **Do not form secondary structures** like hairpins, which can disrupt amplification.

Effective primer design is essential to ensure that the PCR product is the intended DNA fragment without off-target amplification or formation of unintended side products.

Why is Primer Design Important?

Primers directly affect the specificity, efficiency, and accuracy of PCR. Well-designed primers enable successful and reproducible results across various applications from diagnostics to genetic research. Here are a few reasons why primer design matters:

- **Specificity**: Primers need to bind only to the target sequence, avoiding sequences in the DNA template that could lead to unwanted amplification.
- **Efficiency**: Primers with optimal properties contribute to efficient amplification by allowing the DNA polymerase to work without interruption, even over multiple cycles.
- **Consistency**: Well-designed primers can be reused across different PCR setups, ensuring reliable results in diagnostics, research, and even forensic investigations.

3.2.1 Key Considerations in Primer Design

Designing primers requires a balance of several factors to ensure that they function effectively in PCR. Here are the main considerations:

1. **Length**: Primers are usually 18–25 nucleotides long. This length strikes a balance between specificity (long enough to bind only to the target sequence) and efficiency (short enough to avoid secondary structures).
2. **Melting Temperature (Tm)**: The Tm of a primer is the temperature at which half of the DNA duplex dissociates, and it is crucial for stable binding during the annealing step. Ideally, both primers in a pair should have similar Tms, typically around 55–65°C, to ensure they anneal at the same time.
3. **GC Content**: The proportion of guanine (G) and cytosine (C) bases in a primer affects its stability since G-C bonds are stronger than A-T bonds. An ideal primer has a GC content of 40–60%, and often, a "GC clamp" (G or C at the 3' end) improves stability during PCR.
4. **Specificity**: Primers should be specific to the target region, avoiding complementary sequences within the template DNA or themselves.

Otherwise, they may form dimers (binding to each other) or hairpins (binding within themselves), which can hinder PCR efficiency.

5. **Avoiding Secondary Structures**: Secondary structures such as hairpins and primer dimers arise when primers bind to themselves or to each other instead of the template. These structures consume primers and nucleotides, resulting in low yields of the target product.
6. **3' End**: The 3' end of the primer is where the polymerase adds nucleotides. Having a G or C at this end ("GC clamp") increases binding stability. It's also essential to avoid mismatches at the 3' end, as these can reduce primer binding efficiency.

3.2.2 Using Primer3 for Primer Design

Primer3 is one of the most popular and user-friendly software tools for primer design. It is an open-source software available online and can be accessed via web-based interfaces, or users can download it for offline use. Primer3 takes into account various factors (such as Tm, length, and specificity) to design primers tailored to a specific target region.

Steps for Using Primer3

1. **Download Target Nucleotide Sequence:** Go to NCBI Nucleotide database (https://www.ncbi.nlm.nih.gov/nucleotide/). Search for your gene of interest and download the sequence in FASTA format to a text file. FASTA format is a text based format for representing nucleotide or amino acid sequences that is widely supported by bioinformatics tools. The sequence ID starts with a carat sign ">" followed by a unique identifier and the sequence which can be in lower- or upper-case letters. For example, the FASTA for cytochrome b gene of Mithun is:

>JQ404407.1 Bos frontalis breed Nagaland cytochrome b (cytb) gene, complete cds; mitochondrial

CGAAGCTTGATATGAAAAACCATCGTTGTCATTCAACTATAAGAACACTAATGACT
AATATTCGAAAATCCCACCCACTAATAAAAATTGTAAACAATGCATTCATTGACCTT
CCAGCTCCATCAAACATCTCCTCATGATGAAATTTCGGCTCCCTCCTGGGAGTATGC
TTAATCCTACAAATCCTCACAGGCCTATTCCTAGCGATAACTACACATCCGATACAA
CAACAGCATTCTCCTCCGTTACCCATATCTGCCGAGACGTAAACTACGGCTGAATTA
TCCGATACATACACGCAAACGGAGCTTCAATGTTTTTATTTGCTTATATATGCACGT
AGGACGAGGCCTATATTACGGGTCTTACACCTTCCTAGAAACATGAAACATTGGAG
TAATCCTTCTACTTACAGTAATAGCTACAGCATTCATAGGGTATGTACTACCATGAGG
GCAAATGTCATTTTGAGGAGCAACAGTCATCACCAACCTCCTATCAGCAATCCCTT
ACATCGGCACAAATTTAGTCGAATGAATCTGAGGTGGATTCTCAGTAGATAAAGCA
ACCCTTACCCGATTTTTTGCCTTCCACTTTATCCTTCCATTCATCATCACAGCAATTG
CCATAGTCCACCTATTATTCCTCCACGAAACAGGCTCCAACAATCCAACAGGAATC
TCCTCAGACGCAGACAAAATTCCATTCCACCCCTACTACACCATTAAAGACATCTTA

GGAGCCTTGTTACTAATTCTAGCCCTTATACTACTAGTGCTATTCGCACCCGACCTCC
TCGGAGACCCCGATAACTATACCCCAGCAAATCCACTCAACACACCCCCTCACATC
AAGCCCGAATGATACTTCTTATTTGCATATGCAATTTTACGATCAATCCCCAACAAA
CTAGGAGGAGTACTAGCCCTAGCTTTCTCTATCCTAATCCTAATTCTTATCCCCCTAC
TACATACCTCCAAACAACGAAGCATAATATTCCGACCACTTAGCCAATGCCTATTTT
GAACTCTAGTAGCAGACCTACTAACACTTACATGAATTGGAGGACAACCAGTCGAA
CACCCATATATTACCATTGGACAACTAGCATCCATTATATACTTTCTTCTCATCCTAGT
ACTAATACCAACAGCCGGCACAGTCGAAAACAAACTACTAAAATGAAGACAGGTC
TTTGTAGTACATCCAATACACTGGTCTTGTAAACCGGAGAGATGAATTCC

2. **Input the Target Sequence**: Visit Primer3web (http://primer3.ut.ee/) or Primer3plus (https://www.primer3plus.com/index.html) and input the DNA sequence you want to amplify. Paste this sequence into the provided field in Primer3. Make sure the sequence includes the target region for PCR amplification.

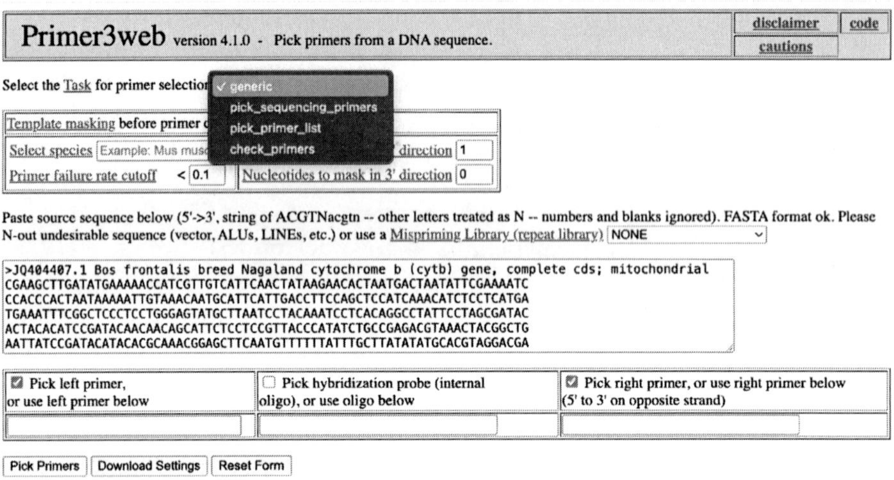

Choose "generic" as this option is used for designing a basic set of primers for a given DNA sequence, typically for PCR amplification. It doesn't have any specific constraints like those for sequencing or cloning, making it suitable for most standard PCR applications.

3. **Specify Parameters**: Primer3 allows you to customise several parameters for primer design, including:

   a) **Primer Length:** Set the range for primer length (e.g., 18–25 nucleotides).

   b) **Melting Temperature (Tm):** Specify an acceptable range for Tm (e.g., 55–65°C).

   c) **GC Content**: Input the desired GC content range (e.g., 40–60%).

d) Product Size: Specify the desired length of the PCR product. For example, if you are targeting a gene segment, you might set the product size range between 100–300 base pairs.

General Primer Picking Conditions

Upload the settings from a file [Choose file] No file chosen

Primer Size	Min 18	Opt 20	Max 25					
Primer Tm	Min 55.0	Opt 59.0	Max 65.0	Max Tm Difference	5	Table of thermodynamic parameters	SantaL	
Product Tm	Min -100C	Opt 0.0	Max 1000(					
Primer GC%	Min 40.0	Opt 50.0	Max 60.0					

Product Size Ranges 100-300

Number To Return 5 Max 3' Stability 9.0

4. **Additional considerations:**
   a) Check "Pick left primer" and "Pick right primer"
   b) Set number of primer pairs to return (3-5 is typical)
   c) Specify excluded regions if needed if there are parts of the sequence you want Primer3 to ignore, such as repeat sequences or highly variable regions that might reduce specificity
5. **Run Primer3**: After entering the parameters, run Primer3 by clicking "Pick Primers". The software will process your input and generate a list of primer pairs that meet the specified criteria.

Primer3 Output

```
PRIMER PICKING RESULTS FOR JQ404407.1 Bos frontalis breed Nagaland cytochrome b (cytb) gene, complete cds; mitochondrial

Template masking not selected
No mispriming library specified
Using 1-based sequence positions
OLIGO            start  len     tm     gc%  any_th  3'_th hairpin seq
LEFT PRIMER        651   20  58.98   50.00    0.00   0.00    0.00 CACGAAACAGGCTCCAACAA
RIGHT PRIMER       865   20  58.98   55.00    0.00   0.00    0.00 CATTCGGGCTTGATGTGAGG
SEQUENCE SIZE: 1246
INCLUDED REGION SIZE: 1246

PRODUCT SIZE: 215, PAIR ANY_TH COMPL: 0.00, PAIR 3'_TH COMPL: 0.00
```

6. **Analyse and Select Primers**: Primer3 provides several options for primer pairs, complete with Tm, GC content, and possible secondary structures. Review these suggestions to select the primer pair that best fits your requirements. Check for any problematic secondary structures and, if necessary, adjust the parameters and rerun the tool.

```
ADDITIONAL OLIGOS
                      start  len     tm     gc%  any_th  3'_th hairpin seq

 1 LEFT PRIMER          502   20  59.05   55.00    0.00   0.00    0.00 CAGCAATCCCTTACATCGGC
   RIGHT PRIMER         670   20  58.98   50.00    0.00   0.00    0.00 TTGTTGGAGCCTGTTTCGTG
   PRODUCT SIZE: 169, PAIR ANY_TH COMPL: 0.00, PAIR 3'_TH COMPL: 0.00

 2 LEFT PRIMER          660   20  59.11   55.00    0.00   0.00    0.00 GGCTCCAACAATCCAACAGG
   RIGHT PRIMER         839   20  59.11   55.00    0.00   0.00    0.00 GTTGAGTGGATTTGCTGGGG
   PRODUCT SIZE: 180, PAIR ANY_TH COMPL: 6.70, PAIR 3'_TH COMPL: 9.19

 3 LEFT PRIMER          233   20  59.17   55.00    0.00   0.00    0.00 AGCATTCTCCTCCGTTACCC
   RIGHT PRIMER         521   20  59.05   55.00    0.00   0.00    0.00 GCCGATGTAAGGGATTGCTG
   PRODUCT SIZE: 289, PAIR ANY_TH COMPL: 3.38, PAIR 3'_TH COMPL: 0.00

 4 LEFT PRIMER          141   20  59.01   50.00   13.34   0.00    0.00 TGAAATTTCGGCTCCCTCCT
   RIGHT PRIMER         267   20  58.76   55.00    0.00   0.00    0.00 CGTCTCGGCAGATATGGGTA
   PRODUCT SIZE: 127, PAIR ANY_TH COMPL: 0.00, PAIR 3'_TH COMPL: 0.00

Statistics
        con   too    in    in   not          no    tm    tm  high  high  high        high
        sid  many   tar  excl    ok   bad    GC   too   too any_th 3'_th hair-  poly   end
       ered    Ns   get   reg   reg   GC% clamp   low  high  compl compl  pin     X  stab    ok
Left   8887     0     0     0     0  3838     0  1300    87     0     0     6    64     0  3592
Right  8883     0     0     0     0  3595     0  1372   110     0     0    11    59     0  3736
Pair Stats:
considered 504, unacceptable product size 494, primer in pair overlaps a primer in a better pair 25, ok 10
libprimer3 release 2.4.0
```

By automating these calculations, Primer3 saves time and enhances precision, helping researchers avoid manual errors and optimise PCR success.

Conclusion

Primer design is a vital step in the PCR process that requires careful attention to length, Tm, GC content, and specificity to achieve reliable amplification results. Tools such as Primer3 streamline this process, making it easier to design primers that are specific, efficient, and tailored to the target sequence. The integration of computational tools has highly improved our ability to evaluate multiple parameters simultaneously, leading to more robust and reliable primer designs.

Understanding the principles of primer design not only improves PCR success but also opens doors to exploring various applications in fields such as diagnostics, genetic research, forensics, and environmental studies. For instance, in veterinary science, well-designed primers are important for applications ranging from disease diagnostics and pathogen surveillance to genetic testing for hereditary conditions in livestock animals. The ability to design reliable primers directly impacts the sensitivity and specificity of molecular diagnostic tests, which in turn affects treatment decisions and disease management strategies in veterinary practice.

3.3 Polymerase Chain Reaction

Polymerase Chain Reaction, or PCR, is a fascinating and essential tool in molecular biology. It allows us to take a tiny sample of DNA and produce millions of copies of a specific region of it. This technique is the foundation of much of modern genetics and biotechnology- from diagnosing diseases to conducting research on ancient DNA. In this section we will break down what PCR is, how it works, the main components, steps of PCR, different types of PCR and applications.

What is PCR?

PCR is a laboratory technique used to amplify a specific segment of DNA. In simple terms, PCR allows scientists to create numerous copies of a particular DNA sequence, making it possible to analyse DNA samples that are initially very small or mixed within complex biological materials.

This technique, invented by Kary Mullis in 1983, relies on the principle of DNA replication. By mimicking natural DNA replication in a controlled setting, PCR can make billions of copies of a target DNA sequence in just a few hours. Mullis's discovery revolutionised genetics, rightfully earning him the Nobel Prize in Chemistry in 1993. Nowadays, the machine for carrying out PCR- Thermal Cycler has become routine equipment in any lab that carries out work in the life sciences such as molecular biology, genetics, microbiology and forensics.

Why is PCR Important?

PCR has become indispensable in many scientific fields that uses molecular biological techniques, including genetics, medicine, biotechnology, and forensics. This is due to several reasons:

- **Diagnostics**: PCR is used to detect genetic material from pathogens, such as viruses and bacteria. For instance, the rapid identification of COVID-19 in patient samples largely relies on PCR.
- **Genetic Research**: In the study of genetics, PCR helps researchers analyse specific genes to understand their function or detect mutations linked to diseases.
- **Forensics**: PCR amplifies DNA found in tiny forensic samples, such as hair or skin cells, helping to identify individuals or confirm genetic relationships.

3.3.1 PCR Fundamentals

Before starting PCR, we need to consider several key factors that will determine the success of the experiment. These are-

Thermal cycling principles: Cycling in PCR is based on three essential temperature-dependent stages: denaturation at 94-98°C to separate double-stranded DNA, annealing at 50-65°C allowing primers to bind to their complementary sequences, and extension at 72°C where DNA polymerase synthesises new strands. We must precisely optimise temperature and duration of each step based on template (sample) characteristics, primer design, and polymerase properties.

Enzyme selection: Taq polymerase, derived from *Thermus aquaticus*, remains the most commonly used enzyme due to its thermal stability and reasonable fidelity. High-fidelity polymerases like Pfu, derived from *Pyrococcus furiosus*, offer superior proofreading capabilities through their 3'-5' exonuclease activity. Modified versions of these enzymes, including hot-start polymerases and blended enzyme mixtures, provide additional benefits for specific applications.

Buffer composition: Standard PCR buffers contain Tris-HCl (Tris is weak base and Hcl is weak acid) for pH maintenance, KCl or NaCl for ionic strength, MgCl2 as an essential cofactor for polymerase activity, and often additional components like BSA, DMSO, or betaine to improve amplification efficiency. The magnesium concentration is especially crucial as it affects primer annealing, enzyme activity, and specificity of the reaction and should be carefully optimised based on reaction setup.

Primer-template interactions: This determines the specificity and efficiency of PCR amplification and is important for primer design considerations such as length (typically 18-25 nucleotides), GC content (40-60%), melting temperature (T_m), and sequence specificity to avoid secondary structures or primer-dimers. The formation of stable primer-template duplexes depends on factors such as salt concentration, pH, and temperature. Thus, careful design of primer pairs with similar T_m values and appropriate spacing on the will lead to efficient and specific amplification of samples.

Components Necessary for PCR

To carry out PCR, we need the following components:

1. **DNA Template**: This is the DNA sample that contains the target sequence you want to amplify. It can come from any source, such as blood, saliva, or tissue samples.
2. **Nucleotides (dNTPs)**: The building blocks of DNA—adenine (A), thymine (T), cytosine (C), and guanine (G). DNA polymerase uses these nucleotides to build new strands of DNA during the extension phase. A balanced mix of these four nucleotides is crucial for efficient DNA synthesis.
3. **PCR Buffer Solution**: The buffer provides the optimal conditions for the PCR reaction, including maintaining a stable pH. It often contains stabilizers and salts to enhance the performance and fidelity of the DNA polymerase throughout the thermal cycling process.

4. **MgCl2:** Magnesium ions are indispensable cofactors for DNA polymerase. They play a role in stabilizing the interaction between the enzyme, primers, and nucleotides. The concentration of Mg^{2+} must be carefully optimized, as insufficient amounts can hinder amplification, while excess can lead to nonspecific products.
5. **Primers**: Short, single-stranded sequences of DNA that are complementary to the ends of the target sequence. Primers provide a starting point for DNA synthesis, guiding the DNA polymerase to the exact location on the template DNA.
6. **DNA Polymerase**: An enzyme that synthesises new DNA strands by adding nucleotides to the primers. The most commonly used polymerase in PCR is *Taq polymerase*, which is derived from the thermophilic (heat-loving) bacterium *Thermus aquaticus*. This enzyme remains stable at high temperatures, which is essential for PCR as certain steps have to be carried out at over 90°**C.**
7. **Nuclease-free Water**: To bring the reaction to final volume.

These components when combined, create the conditions for PCR to replicate DNA effectively and efficiently.

Steps of PCR

PCR is a cyclical process that typically involves three main steps repeated multiple times:

1. **Denaturation (94–95°C):** The double-stranded DNA is heated to a high temperature, causing the hydrogen bonds between the strands to break. This separates, or "denatures," the DNA into two single strands, making the template accessible for replication.
2. **Annealing (50–60°C):** The reaction mixture is cooled to allow the primers to bind, or "anneal," to their complementary sequences on the single-stranded DNA templates. The specific temperature varies depending on the primer design and the DNA sequence.
3. **Extension (72°C):** The temperature is raised to an optimal level for DNA polymerase activity, allowing the enzyme to add nucleotides to the primers and build the new DNA strands. Starting from the primers, DNA polymerase synthesises a complementary strand for each DNA template.

These steps are repeated in cycles—usually around 30–40 times. Each cycle doubles the amount of target DNA, so with each round, the quantity of DNA increases exponentially. By the end of the PCR process, you can generate billions of copies from just a single starting molecule.

3.3.2 Types of PCR

As PCR evolved, scientists developed different variations to suit various research needs. These variations give researchers the flexibility to tailor PCR to specific goals, whether they need precise quantification, RNA analysis, or enhanced sensitivity.

Below are some common types based on their main technical principles and applications:

Core PCR Technologies

- Conventional/Standard PCR: Basic DNA amplification using temperature cycling and a thermostable polymerase to create millions of copies of a target sequence.
- Realtime/qPCR: Monitors DNA amplification in real time using fluorescent markers, allowing precise quantification of starting template amount.
- RTPCR: Converts RNA to cDNA using reverse transcriptase before PCR amplification, essential for studying gene expression.
- Digital PCR: Partitions the sample into thousands of individual reactions to enable absolute quantification without standard curves.

PCR Methods Based on Primer Design/Complexity

- Multiplex PCR: Simultaneously amplifies multiple target sequences in a single reaction using different primer pairs.
- Nested PCR: Uses two sets of primers in sequential reactions to increase specificity and sensitivity for rare targets.
- Touchdown PCR: Gradually decreases annealing temperature during cycling to minimise nonspecific amplification.
- Hotstart PCR: Uses modified polymerases that only activate at high temperatures to reduce nonspecific amplification during setup.
- Allele specific PCR: Uses primers designed to amplify only specific alleles or mutations at a given locus.

Application Specific Variants

- Long range PCR: Uses specialised enzyme mixtures to amplify particularly long DNA sequences (typically >5kb).
- Asymmetric PCR: Intentionally uses unequal primer concentrations to preferentially produce single stranded DNA.
- In situ PCR: Performs amplification directly within fixed cells or tissues to visualise specific sequences in their cellular context.

- Colony PCR: Directly amplifies DNA from bacterial colonies without prior DNA extraction.
- Inverse PCR: Amplifies unknown sequences adjacent to a known sequence by circularising the DNA and primers facing outward.
- Methylation specific PCR: Detects DNA methylation patterns by treating DNA with bisulfite before amplification.

Advanced/Newer Developments

- LAMP: Performs isothermal amplification using multiple primers and strand displacement, eliminating the need for thermal cycling.
- RACE PCR: Identifies unknown 5' or 3' ends of RNA transcripts using adaptor sequences.
- PNAPCR: Uses peptide nucleic acid probes to enhance specificity and enable better discrimination of single base mutations.

3.3.3 Standard Protocol for PCR

Pre-PCR Preparation

- Wear gloves from the beginning of experiment till the end to prevent DNA contamination
- Change gloves if suspected contamination occurs
- Use separate pre- and post-PCR areas to prevent cross contamination
- Use dedicated pipettes for PCR setup and filter tips to prevent aerosol contamination

Storage and Handling

- Reagents, primers, enzymes and DNA template are stored at -20°C
- Thaw components on ice except buffer (room temperature to avoid precipitation)
- Avoid repeated freeze-thaw cycles of reagents by aliquoting frequently used reagents into small volumes
- Keep all components on ice during experiment
- A short spin of buffer, dNTPs, and primers in a benchtop/mini centrifuge is recommended in order briefly to homogenise content and remove droplets from tube walls/caps.

PCR can be carried out either by separate addition of DNA polymerase (Taq polymerase), dNTPs, MgCl2 and buffer to create a reaction mix or with a Master Mix that already contains all required components (except primers). The method of choice can be based on the following pros and cons:

Separate addition

Pros: Customisable; ideal for experiments needing specific adjustments.

Cons: Higher chance of pipetting errors; time-consuming.

Master mix

Pros: Fast, consistent, and less prone to contamination.

Cons: Less flexibility to change concentrations; sometimes costlier.

Steps for carrying out PCR

1. For a 25µl reaction mix with separate addition of components, the typical set up is as follows:

Component	Volume	Final Concentration
PCR Buffer (10X)	2.5 µL	1X
$MgCl_2$ (25 mM)	1.5 µL	1.5 mM
dNTPs (10 mM each)	0.5 µL	200 µM each
Forward Primer (10 µM)	1.25 µL	0.5 µM
Reverse Primer (10 µM)	1.25 µL	0.5 µM
Taq Polymerase	0.125 µL	0.625 units
Template DNA	Variable	5-200 ng
Nuclease-free Water	to 25 µL	-

2. For multiple samples (different DNA templates), it is recommended to prepare a master mix in a single tube that includes all reaction components except the DNA template. This mix can then be pipetted (23 µl per tube) into each PCR tube.
3. Add the DNA sample (5-200 ng final concentration) to each tube separately. This approach minimises pipetting errors, saves time, and ensures consistency across reactions.
4. Make sure to properly close and label the PCR tubes in order to identify the sample that has been added to it.
5. Insert the tubes in a Thermocycler and run it with the proper parameters. Below is a reference for a typical PCR reaction:

Step	Temperature	Time	Cycles
Initial denaturation	94-95°C	2-5 min	1x
Denaturation Annealing Extension	94-95°C 50-60°C 72°C	30 sec – 3 min 20 sec – 1 min 1 – 2 min	30-40x
Final extension	72°C	5- 10 min	1x
Hold	4°C	∞	

Please refer to Appendix C2 for common PCR issues and troubleshooting

3.3.4 PCR Analysis: Gel Electrophoresis

Gel electrophoresis is a fundamental technique used in molecular biology to analyse PCR products, enabling researchers to separate DNA fragments based on size. The process begins with the preparation of an agarose gel, which serves as the medium for DNA migration. Agarose, a polysaccharide extracted from seaweed, is dissolved in a buffer solution (commonly TAE or TBE) and heated until fully melted. Once the solution cools to around 65°C, a DNA intercalating dye, such as ethidium bromide is added to allow visualisation of DNA. The liquid agarose is then poured into a casting tray equipped with a comb to create wells for loading samples. After the gel solidifies, it is placed in an electrophoresis chamber filled with buffer to facilitate current flow.

To separate DNA fragments, the PCR products are mixed with a loading dye, which adds density for sinking into the wells and includes tracking dyes to monitor migration progress. The samples, along with a DNA ladder (a molecular weight marker), are loaded into the wells. An electric field is applied across the gel, with DNA moving toward the positively charged anode due to its negatively charged phosphate backbone. Smaller fragments navigate the gel matrix more efficiently, traveling faster and farther than larger fragments.

After electrophoresis, the gel is placed under UV light for visualisation. The intercalating dye fluoresces when bound to DNA, allowing bands of DNA to be seen and compared to the DNA ladder for size estimation. This visualisation step is critical for determining the success of the PCR and the approximate sizes of amplified products.

Standard protocol for 1% agarose gel electrophoresis

Safety Note: Wear protective clothing and gloves while handling ethidium bromide as it is a known mutagen.

Please refer to Appendix A3 for more information on reagents

1. Prepare agarose gel with the same buffer as the one in the gel tank. This can be either Tris Borate EDTA (TBE) or Tris Acetate EDTA (TAE) (*Refer to Notes at the end*). Add 0.5gm Agarose powder to 50ml buffer in a conical flask and melt by heating for 1-2 minutes in microwave oven. Do not overboil as the buffer will evaporate and the final percentage of agarose will be altered.
2. Once the molten solution reaches around 60°C (you can comfortably touch the flask), add ethidium bromide (EtBr) to a final concentration of approximately 0.2-0.5 μg/mL (usually about 2-3 μl of lab stock solution per 100 ml gel). Adding EtBr to agarose solution at lower temperature ensures that the dye is not over-exposed to heat as it can potentially

cause degradation. Further, in this case where EtBr is added directly to gel, it should also be added to running buffer to prevent staining loss due to diffusion out of the gel.

3. Pour agarose solution into casting tray with comb/s in place to create wells. In case bubbles appear, push it to the sides with pipette tips
4. Place newly poured gel at room temperature until completely solidified. Gently remove combs and place solidified gel in gel box and cover with buffer.

Loading samples and running agarose gel

1. Mix your samples with loading buffer at 5:1 ratio (e.g, 5ul of sample with 1ul of loading buffer). The loading buffer has visible dye to aid with gel loading and gauge how far the DNA has migrated. It also increases the density of the sample causing it to settle at the bottom instead of diffusing in the TAE/TBE buffer.
2. Carefully load DNA molecular weight ladder into first (or last) well of the gel. Load samples in the rest of the wells.
3. Run gel at 80-150 V depending on your sample (*refer to Notes at the end*). Always run from Black to Red. Black is negative and Red is positive and DNA will run to positive electrode since it is negatively charged.

Analysing gel

1. Visualise gel with UV light.
2. Use the DNA ladder as a guide based on manufacturer's instruction to infer the size of your DNA fragment.

Notes

Choose appropriate buffer: Tris-Borate-EDTA (TBE) for higher resolution in separating smaller DNA fragments (<2kb), and Tris-Acetate-EDTA (TAE) for routine DNA electrophoresis, especially with larger fragments exceeding 2kb.

Agarose gel percentage: 0.5%-2%. Lower percentage gels are recommended for larger DNA fragments; higher percentage gel separates smaller fragments better.

Voltage: Ideally 4-10V/cm. Higher voltage (100-135V) is good for fast separation of small DNA fragments while 50-75V provides clear separation of large DNA fragments.

After electrophoresis use PCR product immediately in downstream applications, or store it at –20°C.

3.3.5 Best Practices and Techniques for PCR and Gel Electrophoresis

- Use high-quality, pure DNA template with minimal degradation. DNA must be extracted and stored carefully as the integrity of the starting material has a direct influence on the success of PCR.
- Use fresh, high-quality PCR-grade reagents and nuclease-free water. Contaminated or degraded components can introduce errors and reduce reaction reliability.
- Prepare master mix to ensure consistent reagent distribution across all reaction tubes and reduce the risk of human error during setup.
- Include positive and negative controls for result validation. Controls are essential for interpreting PCR results and identifying potential sources of error or contamination.
- Minimise template DNA contamination through clean workspace and dedicated pipettes. Preventing cross-contamination is crucial for obtaining accurate and reproducible results.
- Use a reliable DNA ladder for gel electrophoresis with clearly defined molecular weight markers. This will allow accurate size determination of PCR products and also serve as a reference point for fragment analysis.
- Prepare fresh, high-quality gel buffer to ensure consistent electrical conductivity and optimal DNA migration. Use TAE or TBE buffer depending on your specific experimental requirements and downstream applications.
- Document gel results carefully, capturing high-quality images with appropriate exposure and scale. Include relevant metadata such as ladder information, stain used, and experimental conditions to support reproducibility.
- Store reagents and samples at recommended temperatures. Proper storage maintains reagent integrity and prevents degradation.

3.3.6 Applications of PCR

PCR has a wide range of applications across many scientific fields. Here's how it's used in practice:

1. **Medical and Veterinary Diagnostics:** PCR has become crucial in diagnosing infectious diseases, such as parasitic, viral, bacterial and fungal diseases. By detecting the pathogen's genetic material in a patient's sample, PCR can confirm infections even when the pathogen levels are very low.
2. **Genetic Research and Mutation Detection:** Researchers use PCR to study genetic variations and mutations that might be linked to diseases.

For instance, PCR helps identify mutations in genes like BRCA1 and BRCA2, which are associated with an increased risk of breast and ovarian cancers.

3. **Forensic Science:** In forensic investigations, PCR is used to analyse DNA from crime scenes, including minute samples like hair or skin cells. The technique can help identify suspects or establish familial relationships.
4. **Environmental Biology and Biodiversity Studies:** Scientists studying environmental samples often rely on PCR to identify and catalog different organisms, from bacteria in soil to endangered species in wildlife studies. This is done by amplifying specific DNA markers unique to each species.
5. **Agricultural Biotechnology:** PCR helps in the development of genetically modified crops by allowing scientists to insert, delete, or analyse specific genes responsible for traits like drought resistance or pest tolerance.

Conclusion

PCR is one of the most versatile and impactful tools in molecular biology. Understanding the components, steps, and types of PCR reveals how this elegant technique amplifies specific DNA segments, enabling scientists to explore, diagnose, and solve complex biological challenges. PCR's power lies in its simplicity and adaptability, and its impact extends far beyond the research laboratory, playing crucial roles in medical diagnostics, veterinary medicine, forensic science, and environmental monitoring. As molecular technologies continue to advance, PCR remains an indispensable tool, enabling breakthroughs in genomic research and contributing to our deeper understanding of biological systems. The technique's reliability, versatility, and continued refinement ensure its position as a fundamental methodology in modern molecular biology and its allied fields.

3.4 Multiple Sequence Alignment of DNA Using MAFFT

Multiple sequence alignment (MSA) is a critical technique in bioinformatics, enabling scientists to compare DNA sequences and uncover similarities, differences, and evolutionary relationships. MAFFT (Multiple Alignment using Fast Fourier Transform) is one of the most widely used software tools for MSA due to its accuracy, speed, and versatility. In this guide, we'll explore the concept of multiple sequence alignment, key factors to consider, how to use MAFFT, and some of the applications of MSA.

What is Multiple Sequence Alignment?

Multiple Sequence Alignment (MSA) is a computational method for aligning three or more DNA, RNA, or protein sequences to identify regions of similarity and difference. By aligning multiple sequences, scientists can analyse evolutionary relationships, detect conserved regions, and understand functional and structural properties of genes or proteins.

In the context of DNA, MSA helps to highlight similarities in genes across different organisms, study conserved motifs and analyse mutations or variations within related species or individuals. These alignments are essential for studying the evolutionary biology, structure, and function of genes.

Why is Multiple Sequence Alignment Important?

MSA is a powerful tool that provides insight into the biological and evolutionary significance of genetic sequences. Below are few reasons why it is essential in molecular biology:

- **Detecting Conserved Regions**: Conserved regions within DNA often indicate important functional sites or evolutionary relationships. By finding these areas, scientists can understand more about gene function and regulatory elements.
- **Detecting single nucleotide polymorphic (SNP) variants:** MSA enables the identification of SNPs, which are single base changes within a sequence that vary between individuals. Detecting SNPs is crucial for studying genetic diversity, understanding population-specific traits, and investigating associations with diseases or adaptive traits.
- **Differences among individual organisms of a species:** By aligning sequences from different individuals of the same species, MSA reveals intra-species genetic variations. These differences can be associated with phenotypic diversity, such as resistance to pathogens or environmental adaptation, and provide a better understanding about genetic factors influencing population resilience.
- **Differences among individuals across different species:** MSA allows us to compare sequences between species, identifying conserved and variable regions. This helps to reveal evolutionary relationships, determine gene function, and understand how specific genetic changes have driven speciation and adaptation across lineages.
- **Understanding Evolutionary Relationships**: MSA reveals how sequences have changed over time, providing information on the evolutionary history of species and how genes have diverged or remained similar.

- **Functional Annotation**: Aligning multiple sequences helps to annotate unknown genes by identifying similarity to known sequences, offering hints about their possible functions.

MSA is therefore crucial in many fields, including phylogenetics, genomics, and evolutionary biology.

3.4.1 Key Factors in Multiple Sequence Alignment

Aligning DNA sequences requires balancing several factors to ensure accuracy and biological relevance. Here are the key considerations:

1. **Sequence Similarity**: Sequences with high similarity are easier to align accurately. If sequences are highly divergent, alignment algorithms must account for variations to detect conserved regions correctly.
2. **Alignment Length**: When aligning sequences of different lengths, gaps are inserted to ensure each base is correctly aligned to its counterpart across sequences. The alignment software should minimise unnecessary gaps for optimal results.
3. **Scoring System**: MSA software generally uses scoring matrices to assign scores to matches, mismatches, and gaps. Higher scores indicate higher similarity, helping identify conserved regions.
4. **Gaps and Gap Penalties**: Introducing gaps compensates for insertions or deletions (indels) in sequences. However, gaps should be minimised to maintain the alignment's biological relevance, with penalties added to discourage excessive gaps.
5. **Computational Efficiency**: The computational demands of MSA increase with the number of sequences. MAFFT is particularly popular because it provides efficient, accurate alignment of large sequence sets.

3.4.2 Using MAFFT for Multiple Sequence Alignment

MAFFT is a versatile, user-friendly software tool designed for rapid and accurate multiple sequence alignment. It incorporates several methods, including Fast Fourier Transform (FFT) to enhance speed and accuracy, making it suitable for aligning large datasets.

Steps to Perform MSA with MAFFT

1. **Prepare the Sequences**: Gather the DNA sequences you want to align. These can be sequences from different species or from different individuals within the same species. Ensure that the sequences are in a compatible format, such as FASTA.
2. **Input Sequences into MAFFT**: MAFFT is available as both a command-line tool and an online web server. If you're using the web server, go to the MAFFT website (https://mafft.cbrc.jp/alignment/server/) and paste or upload your sequences in FASTA format.

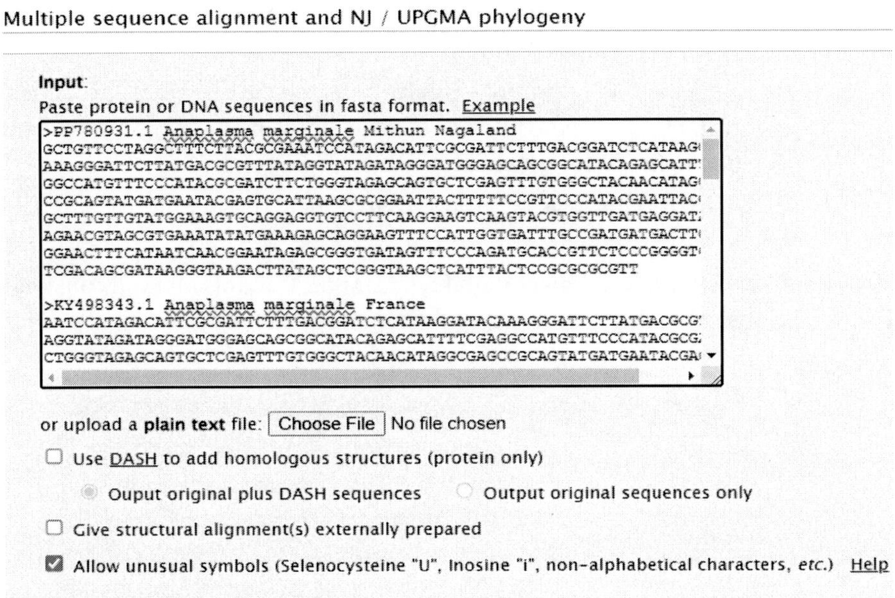

3. Harmonise output sequence order and format

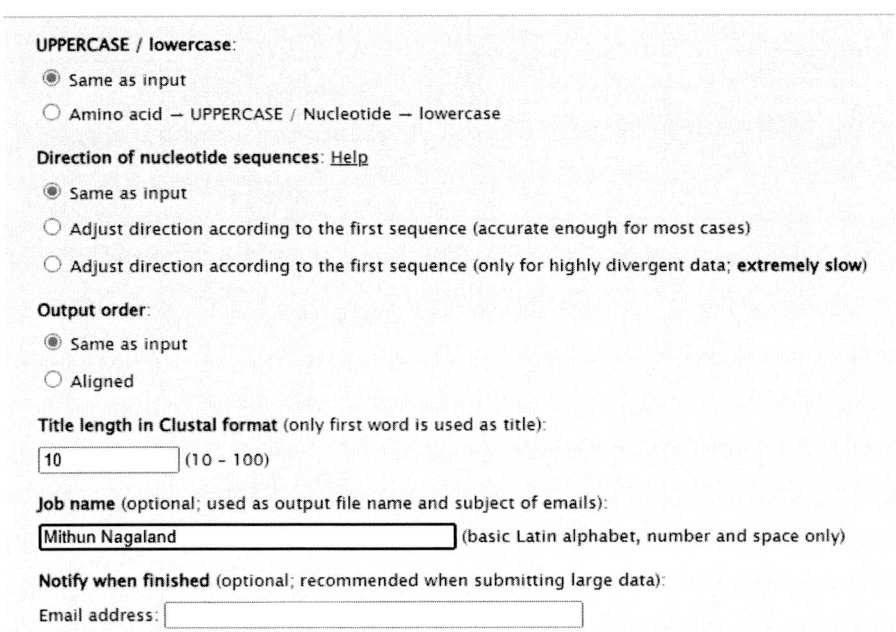

4. **Select Alignment Settings**: MAFFT offers various alignment strategies, with some key options including:
    - **Auto**: MAFFT's "Auto" mode selects the optimal alignment algorithm based on the number of sequences and their similarity. This is recommended for most users.
    - **FFT-NS-2**: This is a fast, progressive method suitable for aligning many similar sequences.
    - **G-INS-I**: For sequences with fewer similarities, this method considers global homology, optimising the alignment for accuracy.

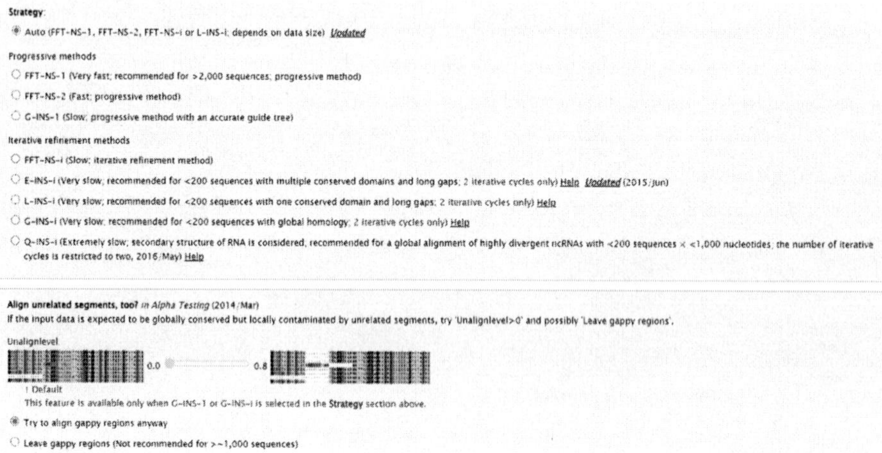

5. **Adjust Advanced Parameters (Optional)**: MAFFT allows customisation of alignment parameters, such as gap penalties or scoring matrices. These can be modified to fit specific research needs, however for general use, the default settings are usually sufficient.

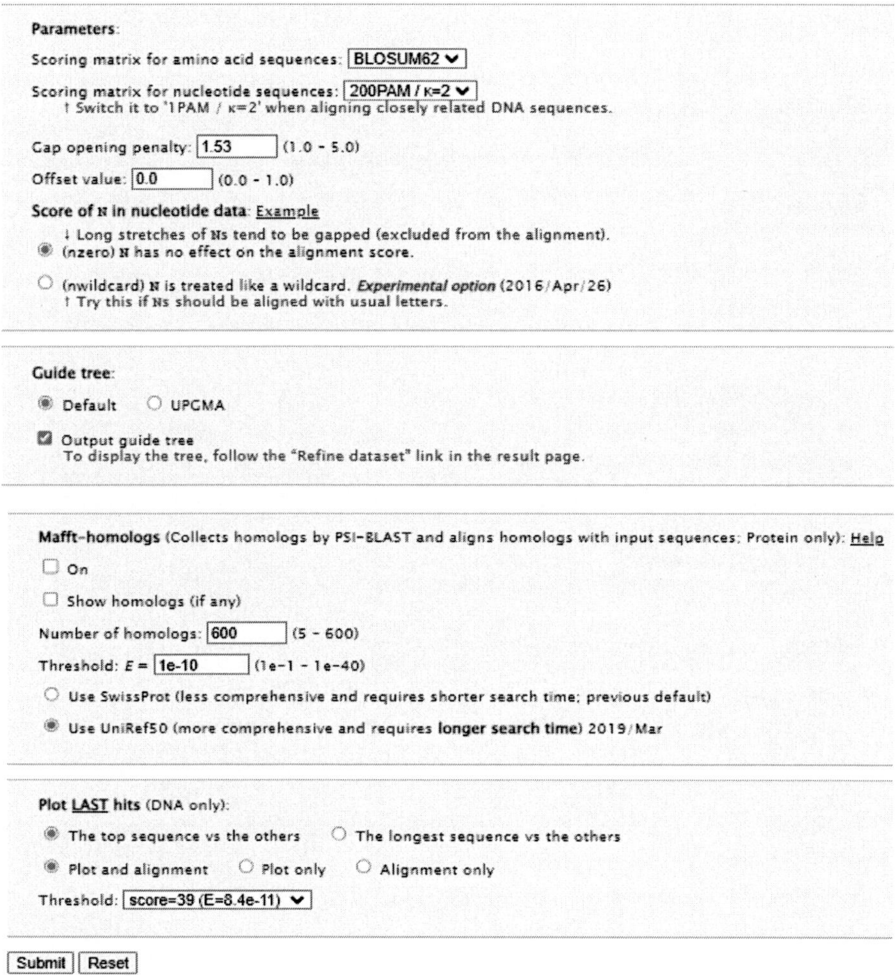

6. **Run the Alignment**: Once you've selected the appropriate settings, run the alignment by clicking on "Submit" button. MAFFT will generate an alignment file showing the aligned sequences, with gaps inserted as needed to maximise similarity.

Clustal format | Fasta format | MAFFT result | View | Tree | Refine dataset | Return to home

View

Reformat to GCG, PHYLIP, MSF, NEXUS, uppercase/lowercase, *etc.* with Readseq

GUIDANCE2 computes the residue-wise confidence scores and extracts well-aligned residues.

Refine dataset

Phylogenetic tree

MAFFT-L-INS-i Result for Mithun Nagaland

```
CLUSTAL format alignment by MAFFT (v7.511)

PP780931.1 GCTGTTCCTAGGCTTTCTTACGCGAAATCCATAGACATTCGCGATTCTTTGACGGATCTC
KY498343.1 -------------------------AATCCATAGACATTCGCGATTCTTTGACGGATCTC
OK322370.1 ----------------CTTACGCGAAATCCATAGACATTCGCGATTCTTTGACGGATCTC
MN284931.1 ------------------------------------------------------------
MT755603.1 GCTGTTCCTAGGCTTTCTTACGCGAAATCCATAGACATTCGCGATTCTTTGACGGATCTC
PP472404.1 ------------------------------------------------------------
OP019038.1 GCTGTTCCTAGGCTTTCTTACGCGAAATCCATAGACATTCGCGATTCTTTGACGGGTCTC

PP780931.1 ATAAGGATACAAAGGGATTCTTATGACGCGTTTATAGGTATAGATAGGGATGGGAGCAGC
KY498343.1 ATAAGGATACAAAGGGATTCTTATGACGCGTTTATAGGTATAGATAGGGATGGGAGCAGC
OK322370.1 ATAAGGATACAAAGGGATTCTTATGACGCGTTTATAGGTATAGATAGGGATGGGAGCAGC
MN284931.1 ATAAGGATACAAAGGGATTCTTATGACGCGTTTATAGGTATAGATAGGGATGGGAGCAGC
MT755603.1 ATAAGGATACAAAGGGATTCTTATGACGCGTTTATAGGTATAGATAGGGATGGGAGCAGC
PP472404.1 -----------------------------------------AGATAGGGATGGGAGCAGC
OP019038.1 ATAAGGATACAAAGGGATTCTTATGACGCGTTTATAGGTATAGATAGGGATGGGAGCAGC
                                                    *******************

PP780931.1 GGCATACAGAGCATTTTCGAGGCCATGTTTCCCATACGCGATCTTCTGGGTAGAGCAGTG
KY498343.1 GGCATACAGAGCATTTTCGAGGCCATGTTTCCCATACGCGATCTTCTGGGTAGAGCAGTG
OK322370.1 GGCATACAGAGCATTTTCGAGGCCATGTTTCCCATACGCGATCTTCTGGGTAGAGCAGTG
MN284931.1 GGCATACAGAGCATTTTCGAGGCCATGTTTCCCATACGCGATCTTCTGGGTAGAGCAGTG
MT755603.1 GGCATACAGAGCATTTTCGAGGCCATGTTTCCCATACGCGATCTTCTGGGTAGAGCAGTG
PP472404.1 GGCATACAGAGCATTTTCGAGGCCATGTTTCCCATACGCGATCTTCTGGGTAGAGCAGTG
OP019038.1 GGCATACAGAGCATTTTCGAGGCCATGTTTCCCATACGCGATCTTCTGGGTAGAGCAGTG
           ************************************************************
```

7. **Review and Analyse the Alignment**: The resulting alignment can be analysed to identify conserved regions, variations, or mutations across the sequences.
8. **Download the output alignment:** Download the aligned sequences in the required format (FASTA, NEXUS, etc.). Keep original unaligned sequences as backup.
9. Use software such as BioEdit (this software can be downloaded from: https://bioedit.software.informer.com/7.2/) for visualisation, which can highlight conserved motifs, gaps, and other alignment features. Trimming of poorly aligned regions can also be done using this software.

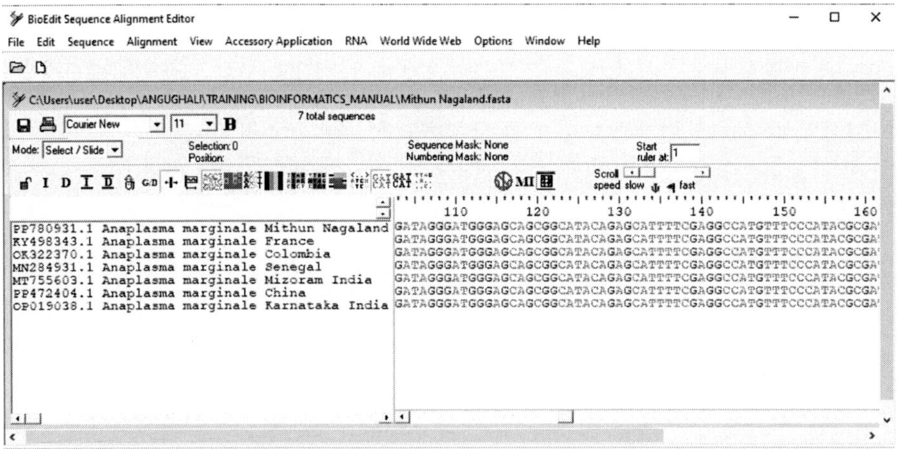

By automating sequence alignment, MAFFT simplifies the process, making it accessible and efficient for a wide range of biological studies.

3.4.3 Applications of Multiple Sequence Alignment

MSA has extensive applications across molecular biology, evolutionary studies, and biomedical research. Here are some ways it's used in practice:

Phylogenetic Analysis

By aligning sequences across species, MSA helps in constructing phylogenetic trees that illustrate evolutionary relationships. Scientists can trace gene evolution, study speciation events, and identify common ancestors.

Identification of novel variants

Identification of novel variants is a key application of MSA. By comparing sequences from different isolates or species, MSA highlights conserved regions and variations, enabling the detection of mutations, insertions, or deletions. These novel variants can provide insights into evolutionary relationships, functional changes in proteins, or adaptations to environmental pressures. This information is particularly valuable in fields such as genomics, pathogen diagnostics, and drug resistance studies.

Comparative Genomics

MSA allows researchers to compare genomes between species, identifying conserved genes or regions that are critical for function. This comparative approach aids in annotating unknown genes and understanding their roles.

Disease Research and Mutation Analysis

In medical research, MSA can be used to compare DNA sequences from patients with different disease statuses, identifying mutations or variations linked to diseases. For example, in cancer research, MSA can reveal mutations in oncogenes or tumor suppressor genes.

Protein Structure Prediction

Although MSA is primarily used for DNA, it is also valuable in studying protein-coding sequences. By aligning homologous protein-coding sequences, MSA can provide insights into protein structure and function, predicting which regions are likely to be functionally or structurally important.

Conservation Biology

In conservation biology, MSA helps to study genetic diversity within and between species, identifying conserved regions that might play a role in species survival. This can inform conservation strategies for endangered species by identifying genetic markers associated with adaptation or resilience.

Conclusion

Multiple sequence alignment (MSA) serves as a cornerstone of modern molecular biology by allowing researchers to analyse DNA, RNA, or protein sequences from multiple sources. It identifies conserved regions that may indicate functional importance, regulatory elements, or structural stability. Further, it reveals genetic similarities and differences that help reconstruct evolutionary histories and relationships between species or strains.

MAFFT (Multiple Alignment using Fast Fourier Transform) is a highly efficient tool widely used for performing MSA, known for its speed and scalability. Its suite of algorithms and iterative refinement methods enables accurate alignments across small datasets and massive genomic or transcriptomic datasets. This capability is highly useful in comparative genomics, where analysing large-scale variations can reveal important mutations associated with diseases, adaptations, or responses to environmental stress.

In phylogenetics, MAFFT helps construct reliable evolutionary trees, shedding light on lineage divergence and speciation. In disease research, it is essential for identifying conserved or variable regions within pathogen genomes, supporting vaccine development, molecular diagnostics, and drug-target discovery. The high accuracy of MAFFT in aligning sequences makes it a valuable tool for genomic and proteomic studies across various biological fields.

Recommended further readings and resources

1. Sambrook, J. and Russell, D.W. (2001) Molecular Cloning: A Laboratory Manual. 3rd Edition, Vol. 1, Cold Spring Harbor Laboratory Press, New York.
2. Soulsby, E.J.L. (1982) Helminths, Arthropods and Protozoa of Domesticated Animals. 7th Edition, Bailliere Tindall, London, 630-637.
3. Urquhart, G.M., Armour, J., Duncan, J.L., Dunn, A.M. and Jennings, F.W. (1996) Veterinary Parasitology. 2nd Edition, Blackwell Science Ltd., Oxford, 224-234.
4. Vandepitte, J., Engbaek, K., Rohner, P., Piot, P., Heuck, C. C., & World Health Organization. (2017). Basic laboratory procedures in clinical bacteriology. In *Who.int* (2nd ed., p. 167). Geneva: World Health Organization. https://doi.org/9241545453

Useful online resources and software documentation

- Primer3 (open-source primer design tool):
  http://primer3.ut.ee/ Primer3 manual
- NCBI Primer-BLAST (checks primer specificity):
  https://www.ncbi.nlm.nih.gov/tools/primer-blast/
- MAFFT (multiple sequence alignment tool):
  https://mafft.cbrc.jp/alignment/software/
  MAFFT online server
- Addgene Protocols (intro to lab bench and basic molecular biology):
  https://www.addgene.org/protocols/
- NEB (New England Biolabs) technical protocols:
  https://www.neb.com/protocols
- Thermo Fisher Protocol Library
  :https://www.thermofisher.com/protocols
- ELISA guidebook (Springer, open access chapter previews):
  https://link.springer.com/book/10.1385/1592590497
- RayBiotech ELISA troubleshooting tips:
  https://www.raybiotech.com/support/technical-support/elisa/

Appendices

A1 Regular Maintenance of Critical Equipment

Thermal Cyclers and Realtime PCR Machines

- Monthly calibration checks of thermal blocks
- Regular cleaning of sample blocks to prevent contamination
- Verification of temperature accuracy using validation plates
- Maintenance of humidity free environment
- Regular software updates
- Documentation of all maintenance procedures

Centrifuges and Microcentrifuges

- Inspection of rotors for damage or corrosion
- Regular cleaning and disinfection of rotors and buckets
- Verification of lid locking mechanisms
- Annual calibration of speed and temperature settings
- Maintenance of proper balance records
- Regular lubrication of moving parts as recommended by manufacturer

Microscopes

- Daily cleaning of objectives and eyepieces
- Proper storage with dust covers when not in use
- Regular servicing of mechanical stages
- Calibration of measuring devices
- Maintenance of immersion oil cleanliness
- Proper alignment and illumination adjustments

Biosafety Cabinets

- Annual certification by qualified technicians
- Daily UV sterilisation as per protocol
- Regular cleaning of work surfaces

- Monitoring of airflow indicators
- Filter maintenance and replacement schedules
- Proper use of UV protection

Autoclaves

- Regular validation with biological indicators
- Maintenance of temperature and pressure gauges
- Cleaning of chamber and gaskets
- Documentation of each run
- Regular safety valve testing
- Proper loading procedures to ensure sterilisation

A2 General Buffers and Reagents

Phosphate buffer saline (PBS, pH 7.4) 10x

(1.7 M NaCl, 0.034 M KCl, 0.1 M Na2HPO4, 0.018 M KH2PO4)

Sodium chloride (NaCl) 80 g

Potassium chloride (KCl) 2 g

Anhydrous disodium hydrogen phosphate 14.4 g

Anhydrous potassium dihydrogen phosphate 2.4 g

Distilled water to make 1000 ml

pH is adjusted to 7.4 with HCl / NaOH.

Reagents for Agarose Gel Electrophoresis

TBE (Tris borate EDTA) electrophoresis buffer 10x stock

Tris base 108 g

Boric acid 55 g

0.5M EDTA, pH 8.0 40 ml

Distilled water to make 1000ml

1% Agarose

Agarose 1g

0.5X TBE buffer 100 ml

Heat the solution till the agarose is dissolved completely.

Ethidium bromide (10 mg / ml) stock solution

Ethidium bromide 10 mg

Distilled water 1 ml

Working concentration: 0.5μg/ml of agarose

Add 1 μl of ethidium bromide (10 mg/ml) in 20ml of agarose solution

Reagents For Faecal Sample Examination

Sodium chloride

Zinc sulphate

Reagents for Purification of Dna From Gel

1M Tris HCl (Tris –hydroxymethyl aminomethane) pH-8

Tris-Base 121g

Distilled water 800 ml

5X TBE buffer

Tris base 54g

Boric acid 27.5g

0.5M EDTA (Ph 8.0) 20ml

Distilled water to make up to 1000ml

Gel Loading Dye(6X)

Tris-HCl (Ph 7.6) 10Mm

Bromophenol blue 0.03%

Xylene cynal FF 0.03%

Glycerol 60%

EDTA 60mM

Reagents for Cloning

Luria Bertani (LB) Broth

Bact. Trypto 1 g

NaCl 1 g

Yeast Extract 0.5 g

Add distilled water to make up volume to 100 ml

Adjust pH to 7.5 by NaOH. Sterilise by autoclaving

Luria Bertani (LB) Agar

LB Agar was prepared by adding 1.5% agarose to LB medium.

X-gal (5'bromo-4-chloro-3-indolyl-D-galactopyroside)

X-gal 25.0 mg

Dimethyl Formamide 1 ml

IPTG (Isopropylthiol-D-galactoside) (1 M)

IPTG	238.3 mg
Distilled Water	1 ml
Filter, sterilise and store at	-20ºC

Ampicillin

Ampicillin powder	100 mg
Sterile distilled water	1 ml
Filter sterilise and store at	-20ºC

Reagents for Competent cell preparation and Transformation

0.1M Calcium Chloride

1M Calcium Chloride (Amresco)	10 ml
Autoclaved double distilled water upto	100 ml
Filtered and kept at	-20ºC

Luria Bertani (LB) medium

Tryptone	10.0 g
Yeast extract	5.0 g
Sodium chloride	10.0 g
Distilled water	1000 ml

Autoclaved before use

LB agar was prepared by adding 1.5% bacterial agar to LB medium

Reagents for Parasitological examination

Eosin Methylene Blue (Emb) Agar

Peptic digest of animal tissue	10.0 g
Di-potassium phosphate	2.0 g
Lactose	5.0 g
Sucrose	5.0 g
Eosin-y	0.4 g
Methylene blue	0.065 g
Agar	15.0 g
Distilled water	1000 ml

pH : 7.2±0.2

Hank's Balanced Salt Solution

Problem: Poor DNA Purity

Solutions:

- Perform multiple washing steps during extraction to remove protein and salt contaminants.
- Consider additional purification techniques like column-based cleanup or precipitation methods.

Problem: Inconsistent DNA Extraction

Solutions:

- Standardise extraction protocol across all samples.
- Use consistent starting material quantities and tissue types.
- Consider using commercial extraction kits and strictly follow given protocol for more reproducible results

C2 Common Issues and Troubleshooting for PCR

Problem: No amplification

Possible causes and solutions:

- Missing component (check all reagents: buffer, primers, dNTPs, $MgCl_2$, polymerase, template)
- Primer degradation or poor synthesis (verify integrity or reorder)
- Template quality/quantity too low (use fresh prep, increase input)
- Annealing temperature too high (optimise via gradient PCR)
- Inhibitors in reaction (purify template or dilute DNA)

Problem: Multiple or smeared bands

Possible causes and solutions:

- Non-specific primer binding (increase annealing temperature, redesign primers)
- Excess primer or template (reduce concentrations)
- Too much $MgCl_2$ (titrate down in small increments)
- Extension time too long (adjust based on product size)
- Contaminated reagents (use fresh aliquots, include no-template control)

Problem: Primer-dimer formation

Possible causes and solutions:

- Primer concentration too high (reduce to 0.1–0.2 μM)
- Poor primer design (avoid complementarity at 3' ends)
- Hot-start Taq recommended to reduce early primer interactions
- Use a touchdown PCR protocol to enhance specificity

Problem: Weak or low-yield product

Possible causes and solutions:

- Low template quantity (increase input or perform nested PCR)
- Suboptimal $MgCl_2$ concentration (optimise in 0.5 mM steps)
- Annealing temperature too low (increase gradually)
- Enzyme activity loss (use fresh or validated Taq aliquots)
- Additives like BSA or DMSO may improve yield in GC-rich templates

Problem: Reproducibility Issues

Possible causes and solutions:

- Inconsistent thermal cycling (check calibration of thermal cycler)
- Pipetting variability (use master mix and calibrated pipettes)
- Reagent degradation (store components properly, minimise freeze-thaw)
- Template variability between preps (standardise extraction protocol)

Further Reading

Diagnostic Parasitology for Veterinary Technicians, 6th Edition by Charles M. Hendrix, and Ed Robinson 2023, Elsevier.

Foreyt WJ. Diagnostic parasitology. Vet Clin North Am Small Anim Pract. 1989 Sep;19(5): 979-1000.

Fundamentals of Veterinary Parasitology by B. R. Maharana, Binod Kumar, et al.

Georgis Parasitology for Veterinarians by Dwight D. Bowman.

Helminths, Arthropods and protozoa of Domesticated Animals by E. J. L. Soulsby.

Veterinary Clinical Parasitology by A.M.Zajac & G. A. Conboy, 8th edition Wiley-Black Well publisher.

Veterinary Parasitology: A clinical laboratory manual (2019) by Kumar, B., Maharana, B. R. Kalyani Publishers, New Delhi

Veterinary Parasitology by M.A. Taylor, R. L. Coop and R. L. Wall.Wiley-Black Well publisher.

Veterinary Parasitology Reference Manual edited by William J. Foreyt, Wiley-Black Well publisher.

Yi-Wei Tang, Gary W Procop, David H Persing, Molecular diagnostics of infectious diseases, Clinical Chemistry, Volume 43, Issue 11, 1 November 1997, Pages 2021–2038.

e-resources

https://www.rvc.ac.uk/static/review/parasitology/index/Index.htm

https://www.sciencedirect.com/journal/veterinary-parasitology

https://www.ncbi.nlm.nih.gov/

https://www.ncbi.nlm.nih.gov/tools/primer-blast/index.cgi?LINK_LOC=BlastHome

https://primer3.ut.ee/

https://pmc.ncbi.nlm.nih.gov/articles/PMC7108329/

Glycerol Saline

Glycerine	50 parts
Saline	50 parts

Autoclave at 121°C for 15 min.

EDTA Solution

To make 500 ml of 0.5 M dissolve 93 g in 400 ml distilled water and bring the pH to 8.0 while stirring vigorously by the addition of NaOH pellets. Adjust final volume to 500 ml and autoclave. Note: it will not completely dissolve until the pH is close to 8.0.

Fixative Solutions for Tissues

10 % Formal Saline: Most useful and commonly used fixative

Formalin	100 ml
Water	900 ml
NaCl	8.5 gm
Duration of fixation	24-48 hrs

Buffered Neutral Formalin (10 %)

Formalin	100 ml
Distilled water	900 ml
Sodium phosphate monobasic	4 gm
Sodium phosphate dibasic	6.5 gm
Duration of fixation	24-48 hrs

Zenker's Fluid: It is good routine fixative with rapid and even penetration in tissues.

Pot. Dichromate	25 gm
Mercuric Chloride	50 gm
Sod. Sulphate	10 gm
Distt. Water	1000 ml

Glacial acetic acid (Add just before use) / add 5 ml to 95 ml Zenker's fluid

Fixation is completed in 12 hrs

Helly's Fluid: In place of glacial acetic acid same amount of formalin (37-40% formaldehyde) is added to Zenker's fluid.

Duration of fixation	6-24 hrs

Bouin's fluid: It is good fixative for demonstration of glycogen and viral inclusions.

Saturated Aq. Picric acid	750 ml
Formalin	250 ml
Glacial acetic acid	50 ml
Duration of fixation	6-24 hrs. or longer

Carnoy's Fluid: It prenetrates very rapidly and gives excellent nuclear fixation with preservation of Nissl substances and glycogen. Being a rapid fixative it is sometimes used when a diagnosis is urgently required.

Absolute alcohol	60 ml
Chloroform	30 ml
Glacial acetic acid	10 ml
Fixation time	1-2 hrs. at RT

B1 Essential Equipment and Supplies Checklist

Personal Protective Equipment

Every veterinarian should maintain a complete set of personal protective equipment, including:

- Heavy duty rubber boots that can be disinfected
- Disposable coveralls or washable laboratory coats
- Disposable gloves in multiple sizes (latex and nitrile options)
- Face masks and eye protection
- Armlength veterinary gloves for rectal examination
- Hair covers when necessary
- Waterproof apron for postmortem examinations

Sample Collection Equipment

Basic collection kit should contain:

- Sterile blood collection tubes (EDTA, plain, and heparinised)
- Vacutainer holders and needles of various sizes
- Clean microscope slides for blood smears
- Faecal sample containers with tight-fitting lids
- Sterile swabs with transport media
- Skin scraping blades and mineral oil
- Biopsy punches of various sizes
- Clean sealed containers for tissue samples
- Sterile syringes and needles

Preservation and Storage Materials

Essential preservation supplies include:

- 10% neutral buffered formalin
- 70% ethyl alcohol
- 10% potassium hydroxide solution
- Physiological saline
- Ice packs and cooling boxes
- Sterile PBS (phosphate buffered saline)
- Sealable plastic bags of various sizes
- Absorbent materials for specimen transport

B2 Required Information for Sample Submission

1. Farm/Owner Information

- Name and contact details
- Farm location and management type
- Veterinarian's contact information
- Date and time of collection

2. Animal Information

- Species and breed
- Age and sex
- Identification number
- Pregnancy status if applicable
- Vaccination history
- Recent treatments

3. Clinical Information

- Present clinical signs
- Duration of illness
- Number of animals affected
- Recent management changes
- Feed and water source
- Previous diagnostic testing

4. Sample Information

- Type of specimen
- Preservation method used
- Collection method
- Time of collection
- Storage conditions
- Tests requested

B3 Blood Sample Collection Issues

Problem: Blood clotting in EDTA tubes

Solutions:

- Ensure proper mixing immediately after collection
- Check expiration date of collection tubes
- Maintain correct blood-to-anticoagulant ratio
- Process samples within recommended timeframe

Problem: Haemolysed samples

Solutions:

- Use appropriate needle gauge
- Avoid drawing blood too quickly
- Prevent thermal shock during transport
- Handle tubes gently during processing

B4 Faecal Sample Issues

Problem: Sample contamination

Solutions:

- Collect fresh samples directly from rectum
- Use clean, dry containers
- Avoid environmental contamination
- Process samples promptly

Problem: Inadequate preservation

Solutions:

- Use correct volume of preservative
- Maintain appropriate temperature
- Process within recommended timeframe
- Use appropriate preservation method for intended test

B5 Issues and Solutions for Various Staining Methods

Staining Method	Issue	Cause/Solution
Leishman Stain	▪ Pale/weak staining ▪ Excessive blue coloration ▪ Precipitate formation ▪ Poor cellular detail	▪ Buffer pH incorrect (should be 6.8) ▪ Insufficient staining time ▪ Deteriorated stain solution ▪ Extended buffer time ▪ Buffer too alkaline ▪ Filter stain before use ▪ Incorrect dilution ratio (use 1:3 with buffer) ▪ Smear too thick ▪ Inadequate fixation time

Ziehl-Neelsen	▪ Acid-fast bacteria appear blue ▪ Excessive background ▪ Fading of stain ▪ Poor contrast	▪ Insufficient carbol fuchsin heating ▪ Incomplete decolorisation ▪ Reduce acid-alcohol decolorisation time ▪ Improper storage (exposure to light) ▪ Old reagents ▪ Adjust methylene blue counterstaining time
Modified Z-N	▪ Weak oocyst staining ▪ Over-decolorisation ▪ Poor internal structure visibility	▪ Increase carbol fuchsin staining time ▪ Reduce acid-alcohol exposure ▪ Switch to 1% sulfuric acid ▪ Adjust counterstain timing ▪ Check smear thickness
Giemsa	▪ Granular precipitate ▪ Poor cell differentiation ▪ Uneven staining ▪ Green metallic sheen	▪ Filter before use ▪ Use fresh working solution ▪ Check buffer pH (6.8-7.2) ▪ Adjust staining time ▪ Ensure level staining surface ▪ Apply stain uniformly ▪ Remove residual oil immersion ▪ Complete drying before mounting
D'Antoni	▪ Poor trophozoite visualisation ▪ Rapid stain deterioration ▪ Crystallisation	▪ Use fresh samples ▪ Check iodine concentration ▪ Store in amber bottle ▪ Prepare fresh weekly ▪ Filter before use ▪ Store at 15-25°C
Modified Wright	▪ Poor nuclear detail ▪ Cytoplasmic basophilia ▪ Stain precipitation	▪ Check fixation time ▪ Verify buffer pH ▪ Reduce staining time ▪ Adjust buffer concentration ▪ Filter before use ▪ Check storage conditions
Lactophenol Cotton Blue	▪ Air bubbles ▪ Crystal formation ▪ Fading fungal structures ▪ Poor internal structure visibility	▪ Apply coverslip at 45° angle ▪ Use appropriate stain volume ▪ Filter solution ▪ Check storage temperature ▪ Seal coverslip edges ▪ Adjust stain concentration ▪ Check mounting technique

B6 Common Issues and Troubleshooting for ELISA

Problem: Non-specific Binding/High Background

Solutions:

- Optimise blocking buffer concentration and incubation time
- Increase washing frequency and duration between steps
- Verify antibody specificity and cross-reactivity
- Use fresh, properly filtered buffers
- Ensure proper storage conditions for all reagents
- Check plate for scratches or contamination

Problem: Weak or No Signal

Solutions:

- Verify protein/antigen coating concentration
- Confirm primary and secondary antibody concentrations
- Check substrate freshness and proper storage
- Ensure correct pH of coating buffer
- Validate enzyme conjugate activity
- Monitor incubation temperature and duration

Problem: Poor Reproducibility Between Wells

Solutions:

- Maintain consistent incubation times for all wells
- Ensure uniform temperature across the plate
- Use calibrated pipettes and proper technique
- Standardise washing procedure for all wells
- Verify proper mixing of reagents before use
- Avoid edge effects by filling outer wells with buffer

Problem: Inconsistent Standard Curve

Solutions:

- Prepare fresh standards for each assay run
- Use consistent dilution technique
- Allow all reagents to reach room temperature
- Verify proper storage of standard stock solution
- Follow consistent plate layout between assays
- Use appropriate curve-fitting model

Problem: Edge Effects

Solutions:

- Pre-incubate plates at assay temperature
- Fill outer wells with buffer only

- Avoid temperature gradients during incubation
- Use appropriate plate sealers
- Handle plates carefully to avoid vibration

Problem: Substrate Development Issues

Solutions:

- Check substrate storage conditions
- Verify enzyme conjugate activity
- Optimise substrate incubation time
- Protect light-sensitive substrates
- Use clean glassware for substrate preparation
- Monitor room temperature during development

C1 Common Issues and Troubleshooting for DNA Extraction

Problem: Low DNA Yield

Solutions:

- Ensure thorough cell lysis using an appropriate lysis buffer. Select a lysis buffer compatible with your sample type (e.g., CTAB for plant tissues, proteinase K for animal cells).
- Optimise DNA precipitation and recovery steps. Use cold ethanol or isopropanol, centrifuge at high speeds, and carefully remove supernatant to maximise DNA collection.
- Use ice-cold reagents. Cold temperatures help prevent DNA degradation and improve precipitation efficiency.

Problem: DNA Contamination

Solutions:

- Use sterile, DNase-free equipment and consumables. Contamination can introduce foreign genetic material and compromise experimental results.
- Implement rigorous cleaning protocols for workspaces and pipettes. Regular decontamination with bleach or UV irradiation reduces the risk of exogenous DNA introduction.
- Wear clean gloves and change them frequently during extraction process.

Problem: DNA Degradation

Solutions:

- Store DNA samples at appropriate temperatures (-20°C for short-term, -80°C for long-term storage).
- Minimise repeated freeze-thaw cycles which can fragment DNA molecules.
- Use RNA/DNA stabilisation reagents during extraction and storage.

Unit I

Sodium chloride	16.0 g
Potassium chloride	0.80 g
Magnesium sulphate, 7 H2 0	0.40 g
Calcium chloride dehydrate	0.343 g
Distilled water	200 ml

Unit II

Di- sodium hydrogen phosphate	0.297 g
Potassium hydrogen phosphate	0.12 g
Dextrose	4.0 g
Phonol red (0.4%)	10.0 ml
Distilled water	200 ml

Unit III

Sodium biocarbonate	2.7 g
Distilled water	100 ml

Working Solution

Unit l	10.0 ml
Unit ll	10.0 ml
Unit lll	2.5 ml
Distilled water	77.5 ml

Normal Saline Solution

Sodium chloride	8.0 g
Distilled water	1000 ml

Nutrient Agar

Beef extract	10.0 g
Peptone	10.0 g
Sodium chloride	5.0 g
Agar	20.0 g
Distilled water	1000 ml

pH: 7.2±0.2

pH: 7.3± 0.1

Phosphate Buffer

Solution A 0.2 M monobasic sodium phosphate

Sodium di-hydrogen phosphate dehydrate	31.2 g
Distilled water	upto 1000 ml

Solution B 0.2M dibasic sodium phosphate

Di-sodium hydrogen phosphate	28.39 g
Distilled water	up to 1000 ml

Final solution

Solution A	39 ml
Solution B	61 ml

pH: 7.0

Phosphate Buffer Saline

Sodium chloride	8.0 g
Potassium chloride	0.20 g
Di-sodium hydrogen phosphate	1.15 g
Potassium di-hydrogen phosphate	0.20 g
Distilled water	1000 ml

pH : 7.2

Lugol's Iodine

Stock solution

Iodine	5.0 g
Pot. Iodide	10.0 g
Distilled water	100 ml

Working solution

For use dilute 1:5 with distilled water

Methiyl Red Indicator

Methyl red	0.1 g
Alcohol (95%)	300 ml
Distilled water	200 ml

Phosphate buffered glycerine

PBS (pH 7.4)	50 parts
Glycerin	50 parts

Parasites: At a glance

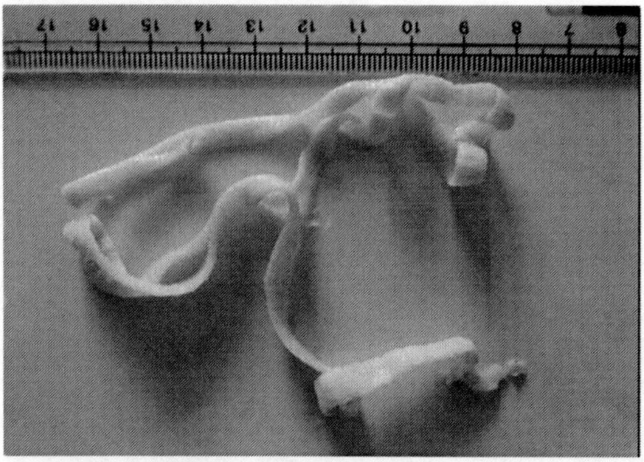

Tape worm (Taenia)

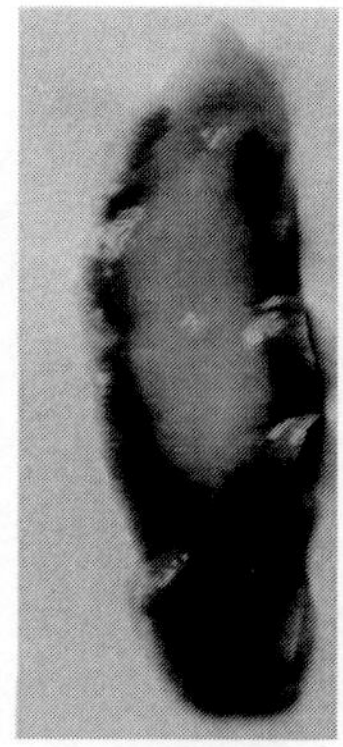

Fluke (Fasciola)

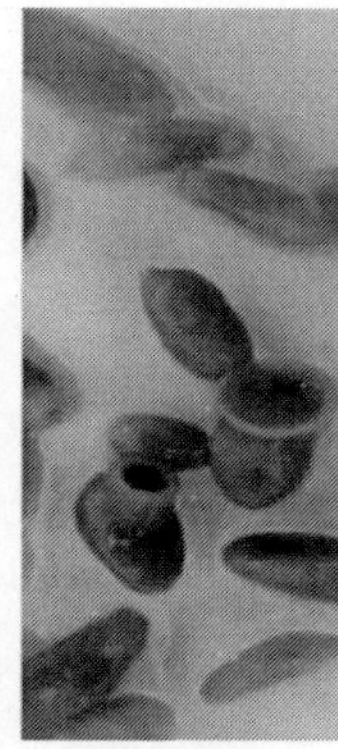

Amphistomes

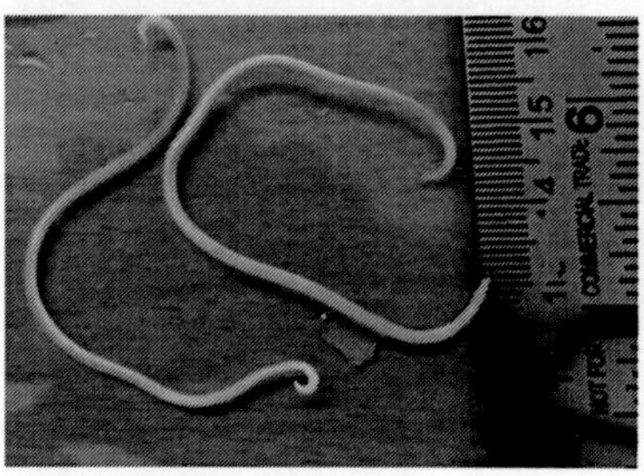

Roundworm (Toxocara)

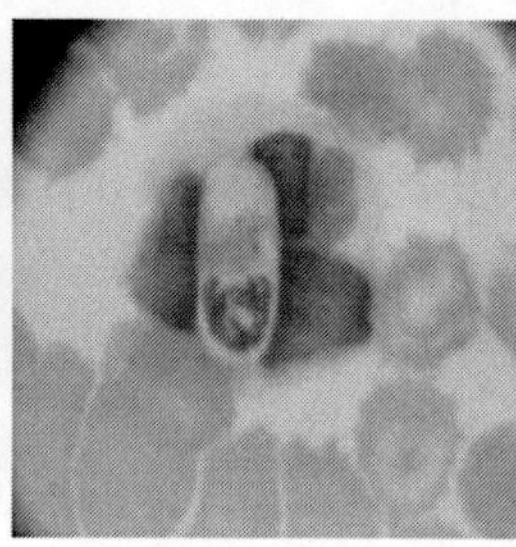

Hepatozoon in neutrophil

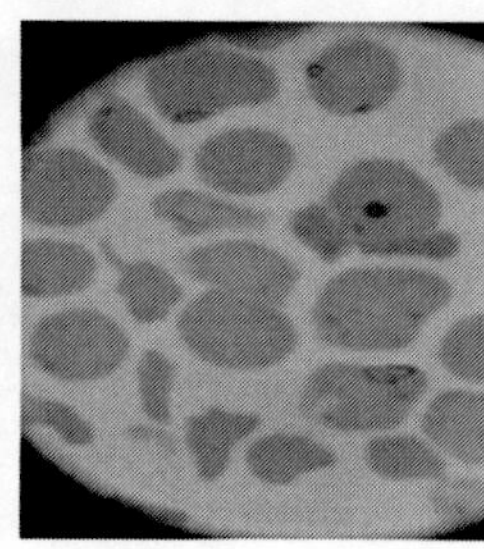

Anaplasma in RBCs

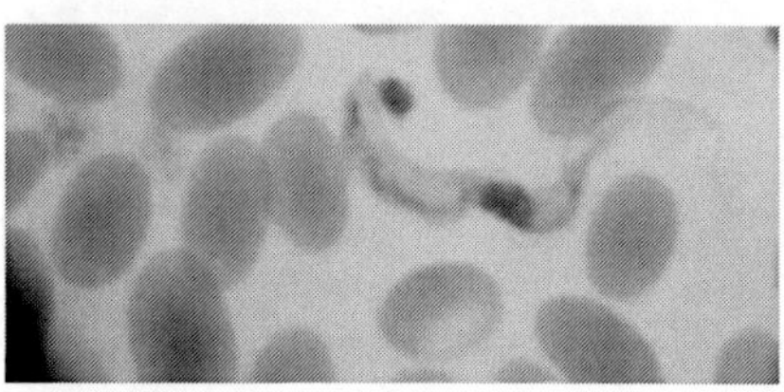

Trypanosoma in blood plasma

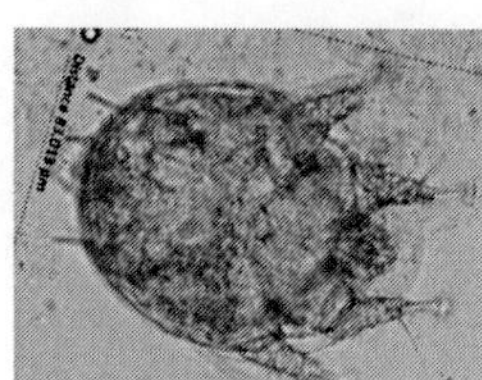

Mites (*Sarcoptes*)

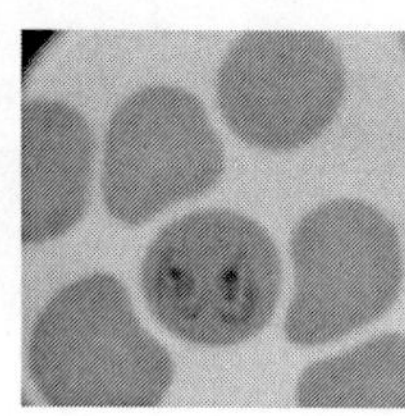

Babesia in RBC

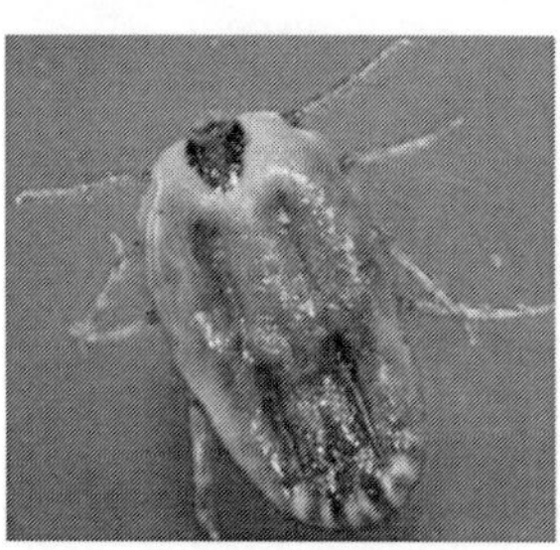

Hard tick (Rhipicephalus microplus) Female

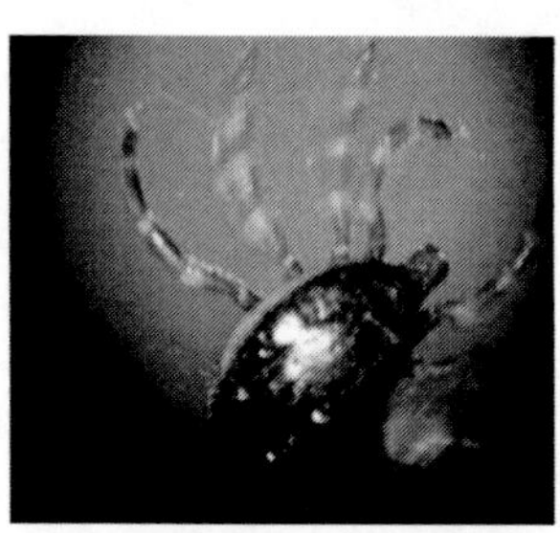

Hard tick (*Hyalomma* spp.) Male

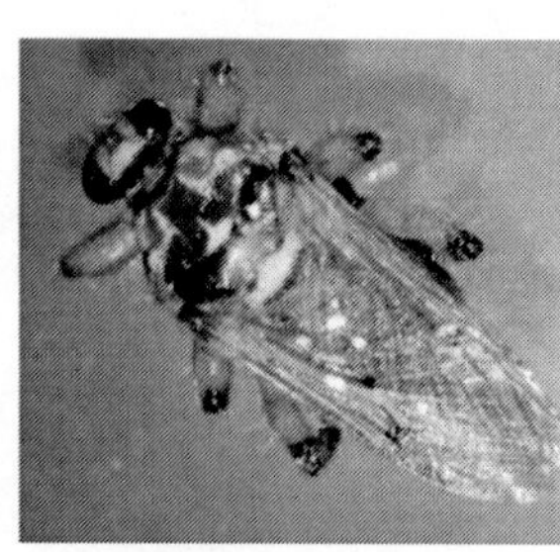

Flies (*Hippobosca*)

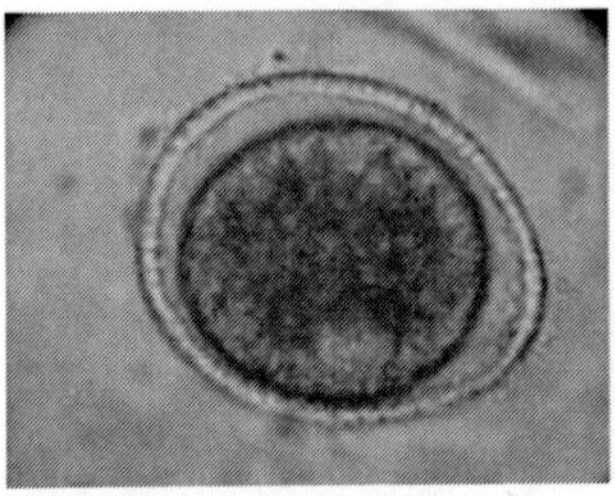
Ascarid eggs (Toxocara)

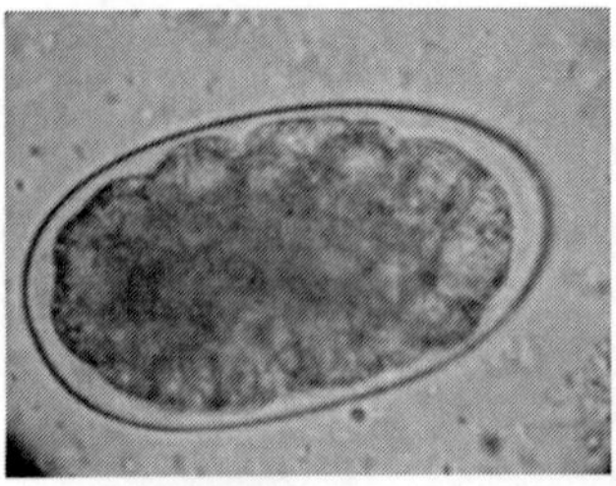
Strongyle eggs

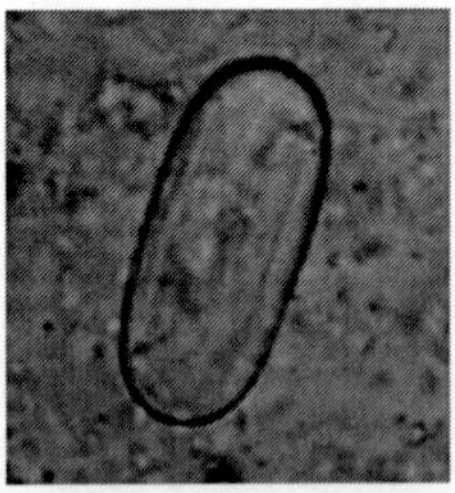
Spirurid egg (*Spirocerca*)

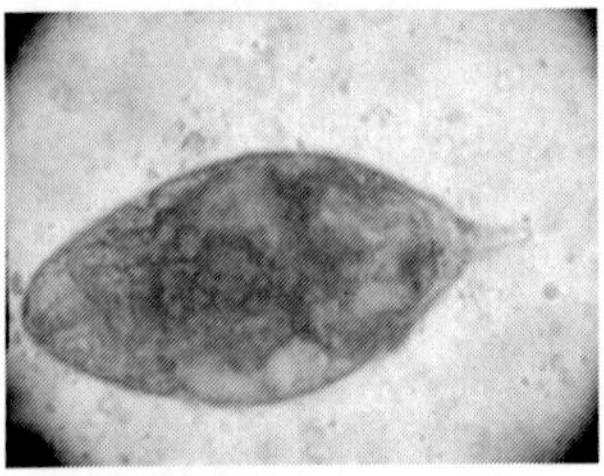
Pseudoparasite

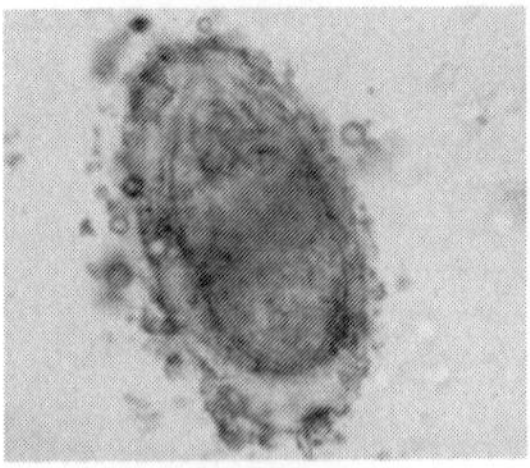
Schis tosoma egg

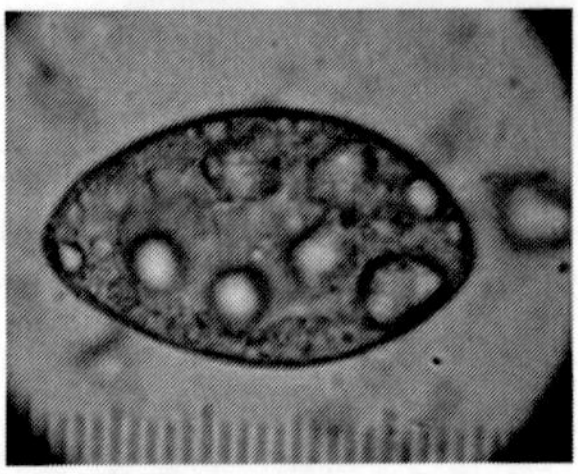
Egg (*Spirometra*)

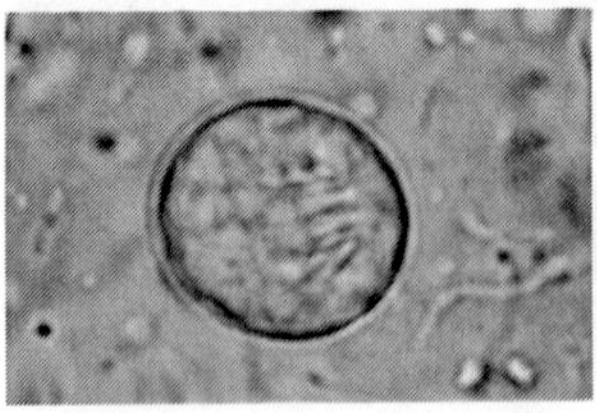
Egg (*Taenia*)

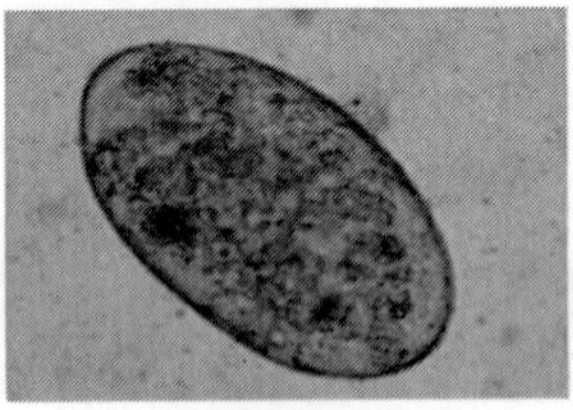
Egg (Amphistome)

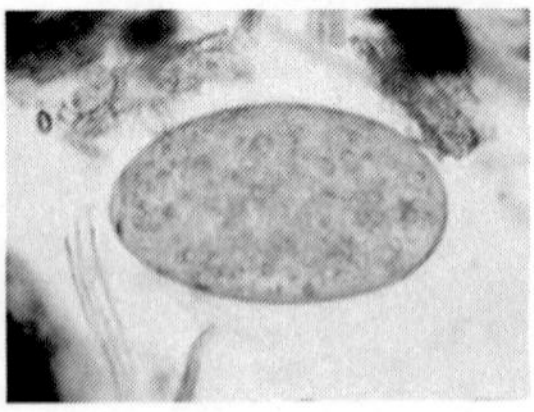
Egg (*Fasciola*)

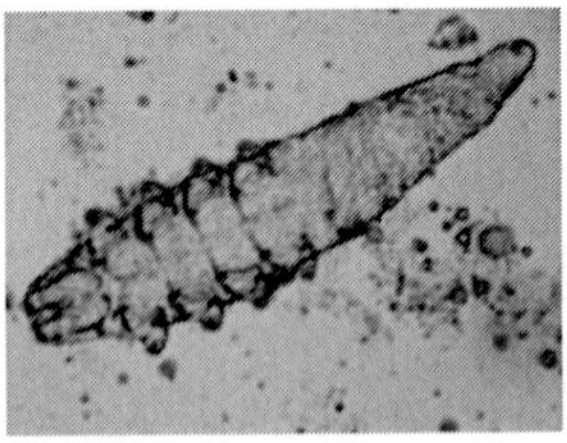
Adult mite (*Demodex*)

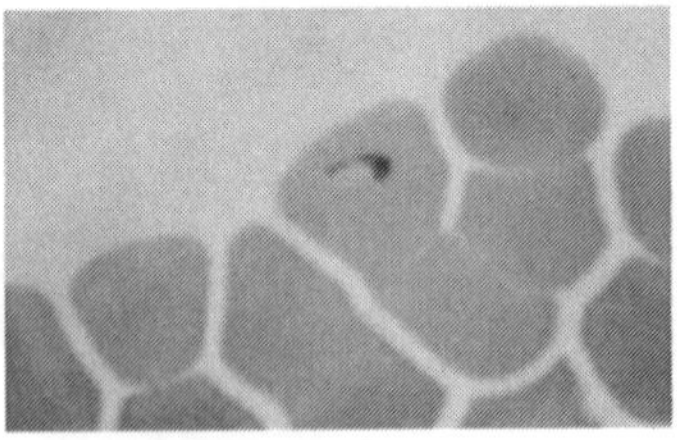
Theileria in RBC

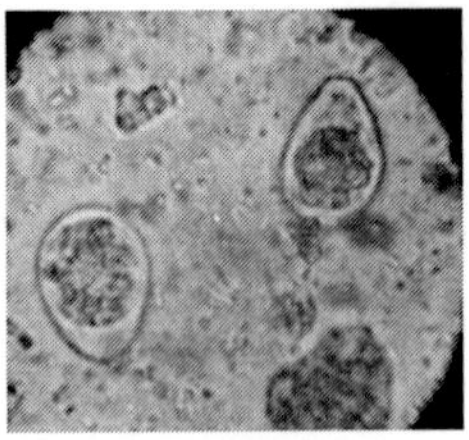
Coccidian oocyst (unsporulated)

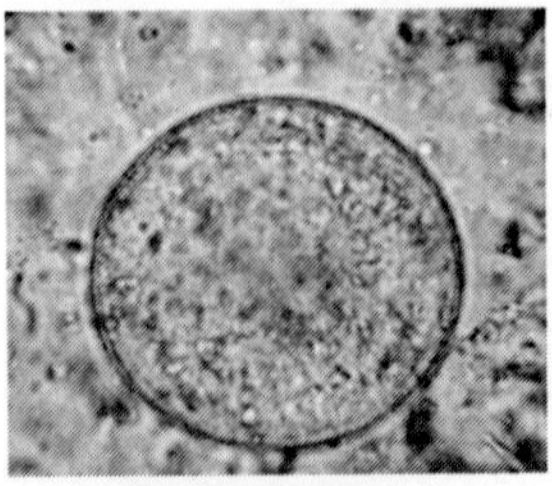
Cyst (*Buxtonella*)

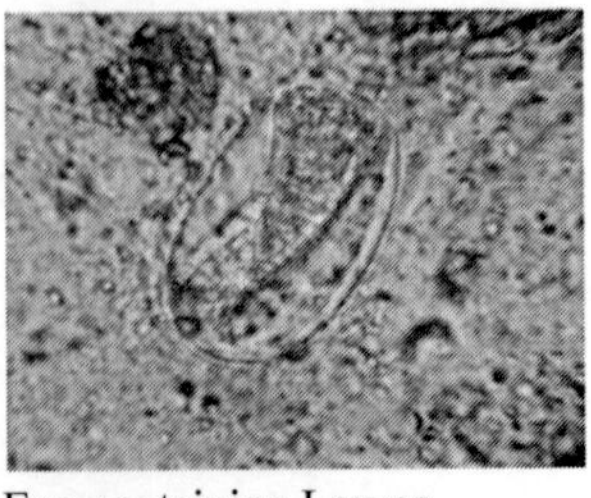
Egg containing Larvae (Strongyloides)

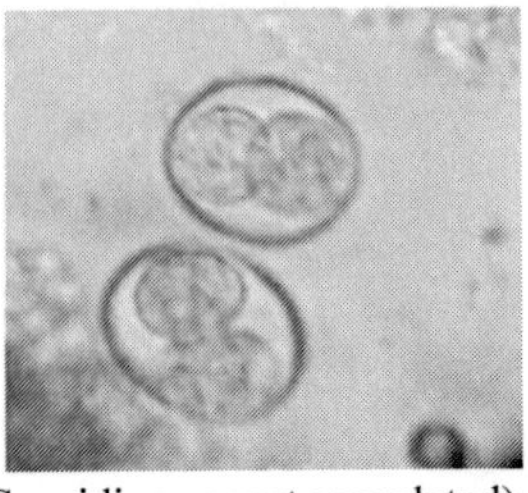
Coccidian oocyst sporulated)

Guide for Interpretation of Worm Egg Count (EPG)

Hosts	Parasite	epg	severity
Equine	Nematode	500	Mild
		800-1000	Moderate
		1500-2000	Severe
Sheep	Nematode	2000-6000	Severe though depend on spp. of Worm
Cattle		100-300	Mild
		300-600	Moderate
		600-800	Severe
Trematode	Cattle	50-100	mild
		100-200	Moderate
		200-400	Severe
	Sheep/goats	300-600	pathogenic

Hosts	Parasite	Light	Moderate	Severe
Cattle	Mixed	-	200-700	> 700
	Haemonchus	200	200-500	> 500
	Oestertagia	150	150-500	>500
	Tricostrongylus axei	50	50-300	>300
	Trichostrongylus spp	-	-	>500
	Bunostomum spp	20	20-100	>100
	Cooperia spp	500	500-3000	>3000
	C. puntata	50	50-200	>200
	Oesophagostomum	50-150	150-500	>500
	Fasciola spp	50-150	150-500	>500
	Fasciola	60-200	200-500	>500

Worm spp:

Hosts	Parasites	Light	Moderate	Heavy
Sheep and goat	Mixed infection	______	1000	2000
	Mixed infection absent	________	500	1000
	Haemonchus	100-2,500	2500-8000	8000 and above
	Oestertagia	50-200	200-2000	2000 and above
	Trichostrongylus axei	____	____	3000 and above
	Trichostrongylus. Spp	100-500	500-2000	2000 and above
	Nematodirus	50-100	100-600	600 and above
	Strongyloides	____	____	10,000 and above
	Gaigeria	100-200	200-800	800 and above
	Chabertia	_____	_____	1000 and above
Sheep and goat	*Oesophagostomum*	100-1000	1000-2000	3000 and above

(Ref.: Rathore, V. S. and Sengar, Y. S. (2005). Diagnostic Parasitology (for Pathologists, Parasitologist, Physiologists, Lab. Technicians) Pointer Publisher, Jeypore. Pp: 39-40).

Colour Plates

Chapter 1: Laboratory Fundamentals and Safety Practices

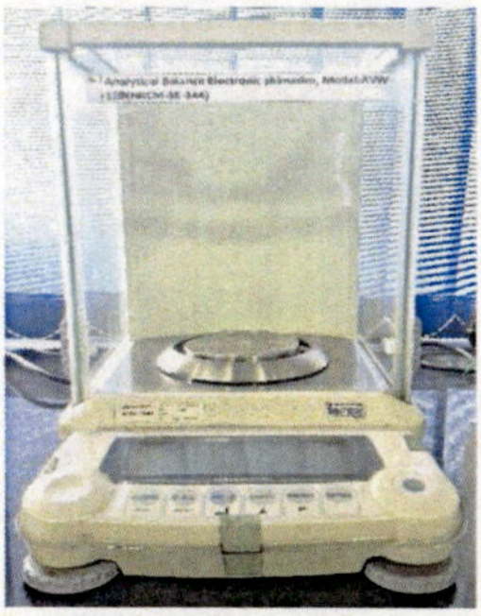

Fig. 1: Analytical electronic balance

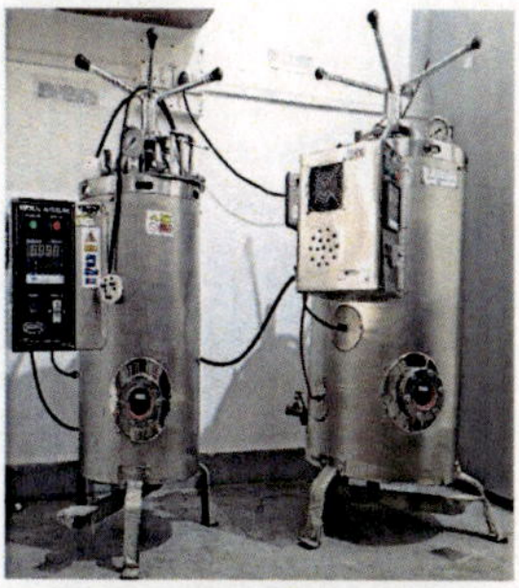

Fig. 2: Autoclaves (vertical)

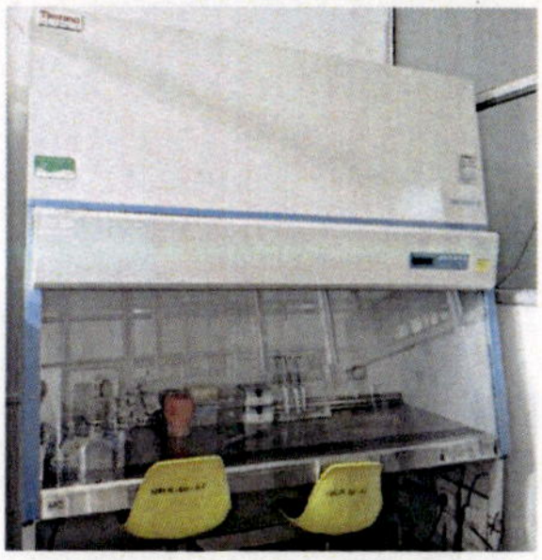

Fig. 3: Biosafety cabinet

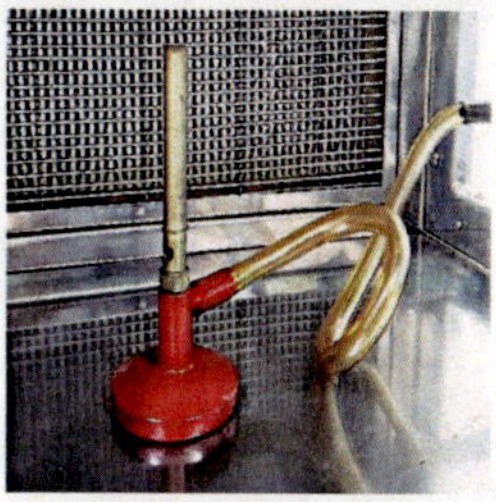

Fig. 4: Burner

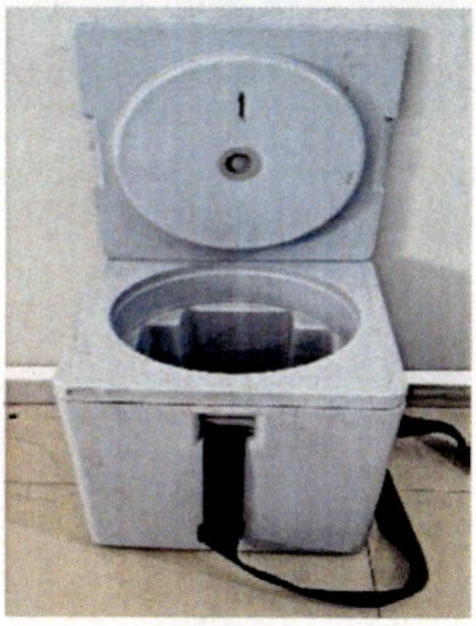

Fig. 5: Cold chain box

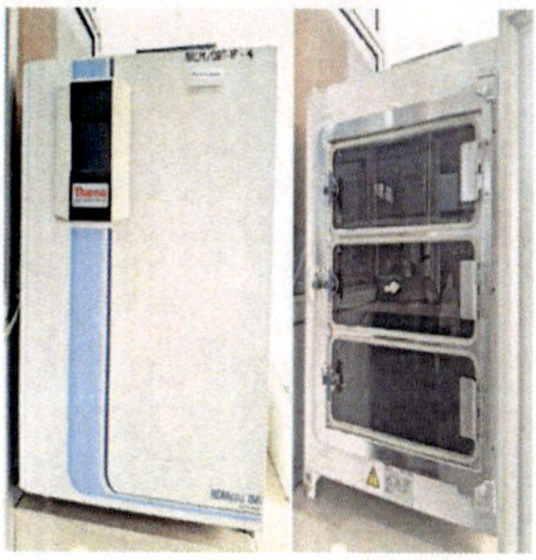

Fig. 6: CO_2 incubator

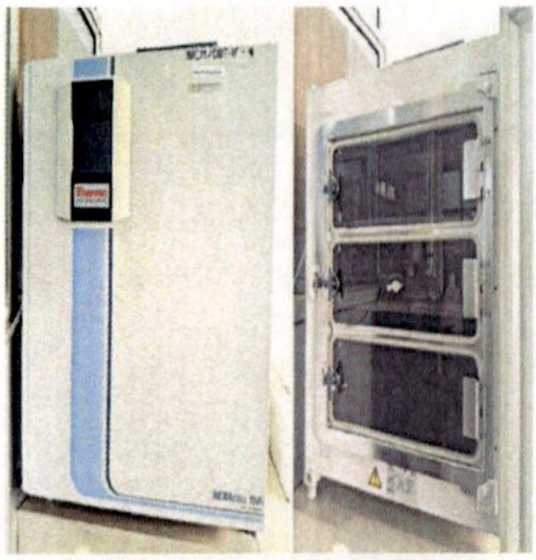

Fig. 6: CO_2 incubator

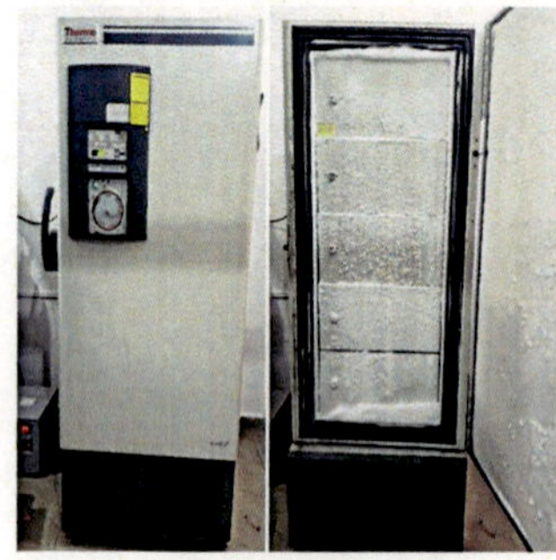

Fig. 7: Deep freezer (-80°C)

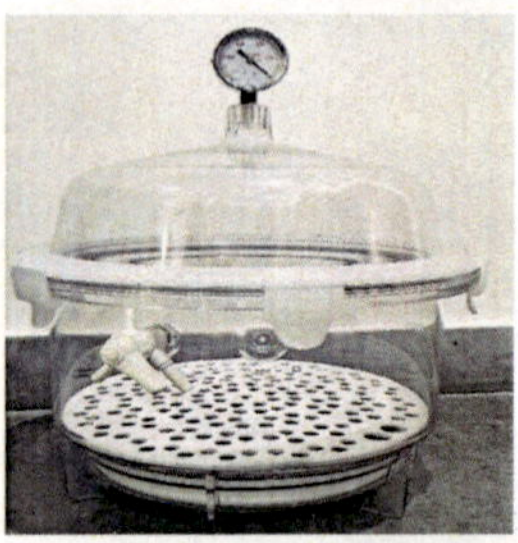

Fig. 8: Dessicator

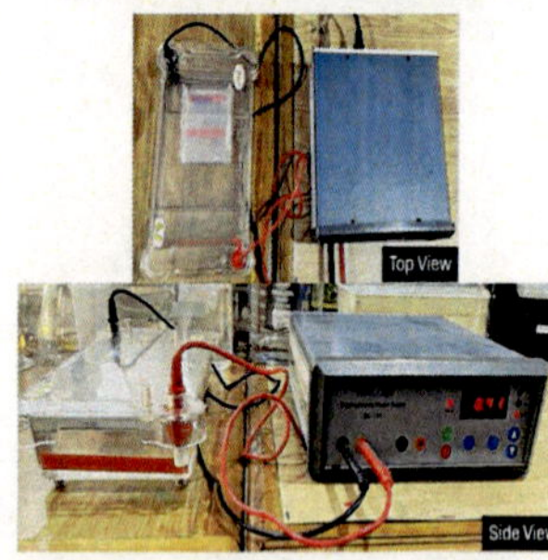

Fig. 9: Electrophoresis unit

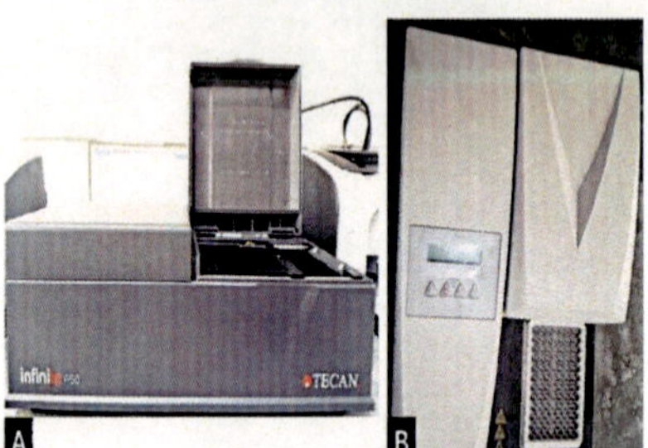

Fig. 10: ELISA reader

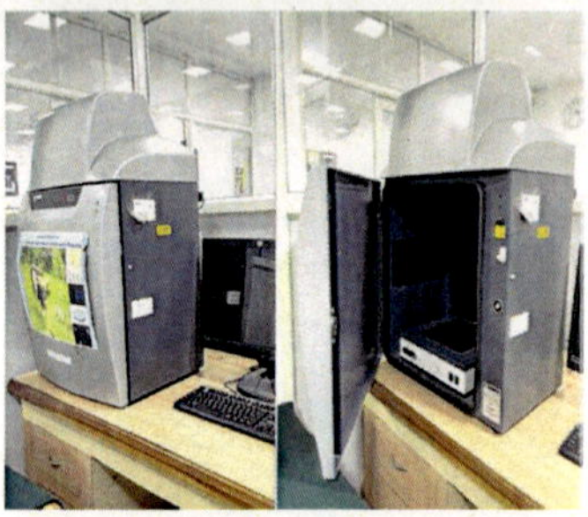

Fig. 11: Gel documentation system

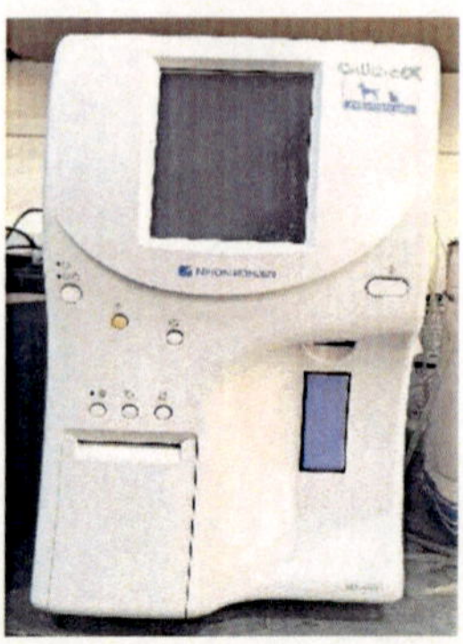

Fig. 12: Haematology analyser

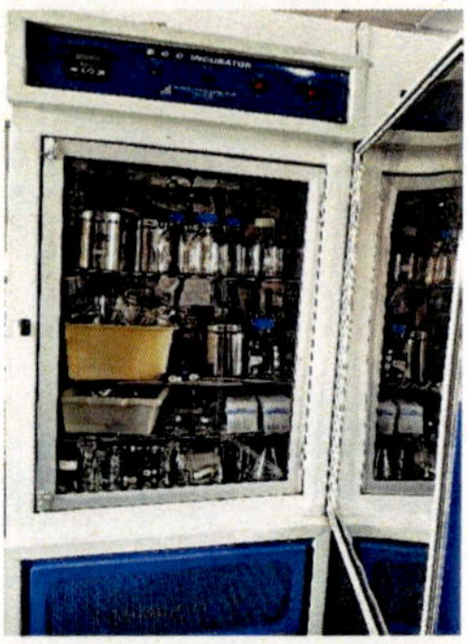

Fig. 13: Hot air oven

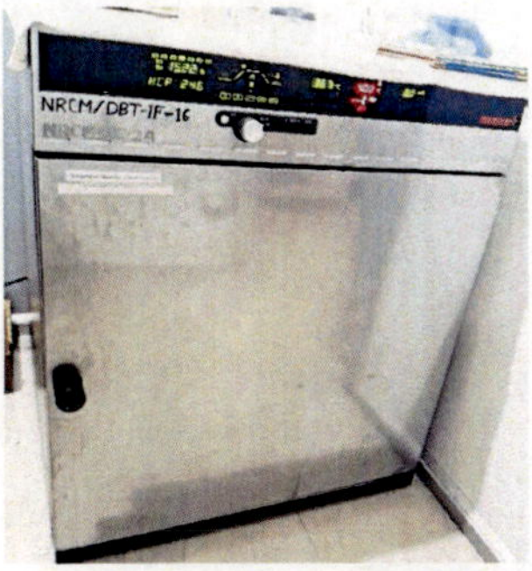

Fig. 14: Incubator

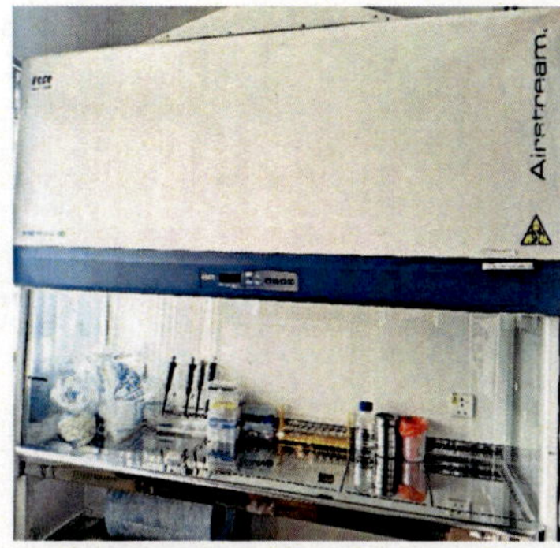

Fig. 15: Laminar hood with UV light

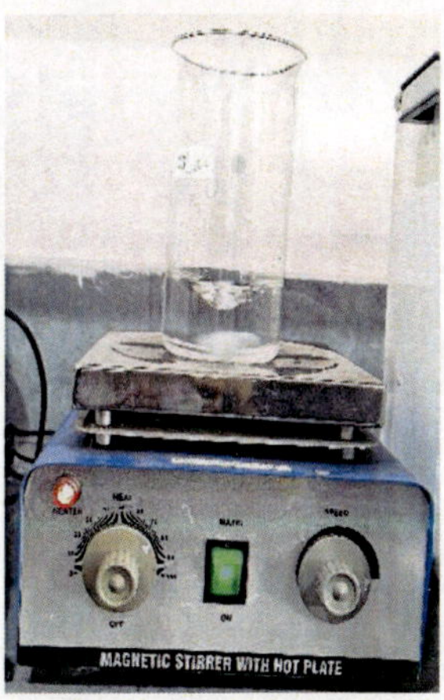

Fig. 16: Magnetic stirrer

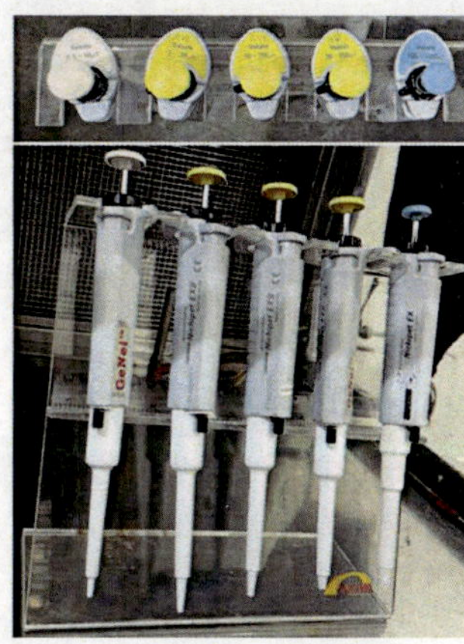

Fig. 17: Micropipette

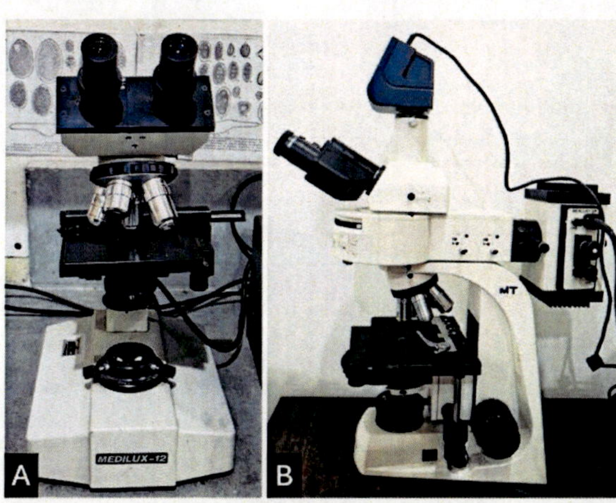

Fig. 18: Microscope

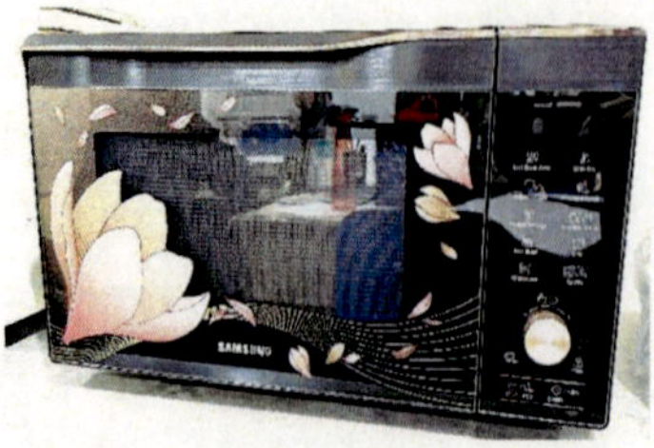

Fig. 19: Microwave oven

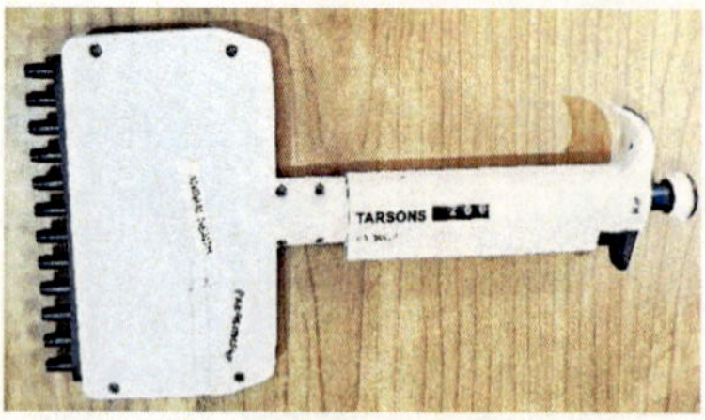

Fig. 20: Multi-channel pipette

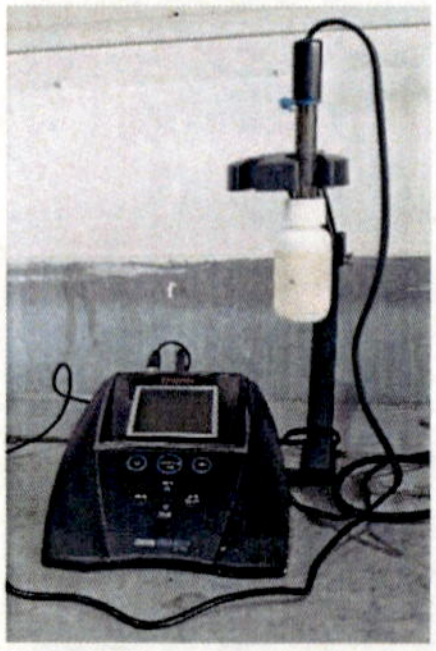

Fig. 21: pH meter

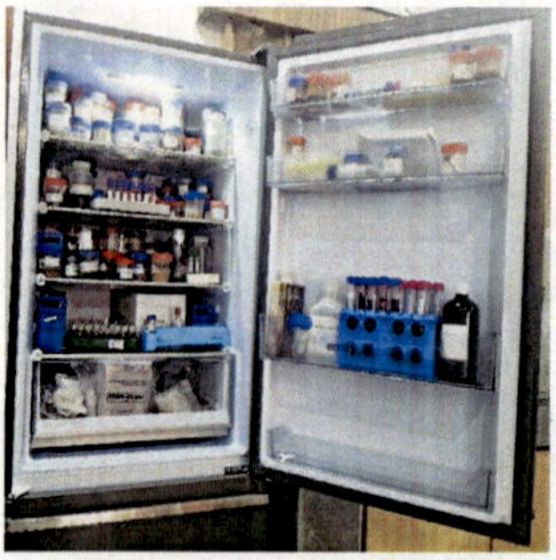

Fig. 22: Refrigerator

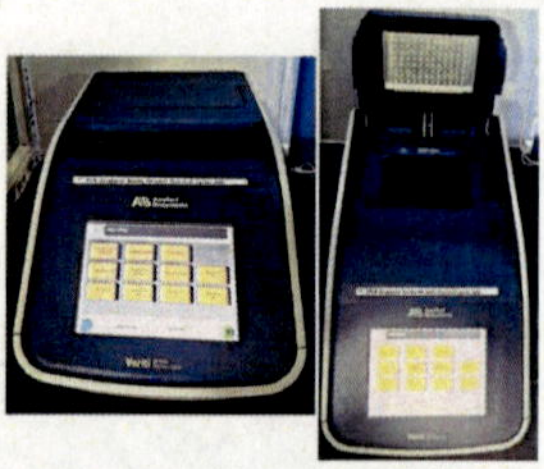

Fig. 23: Thermal cycler

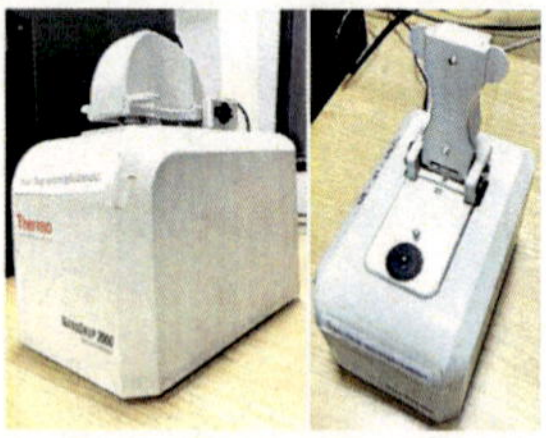

Fig. 24: UV spectrophotometer

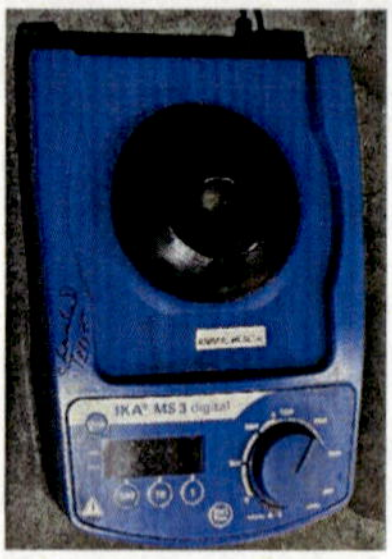

Fig. 25: Vortex mixer

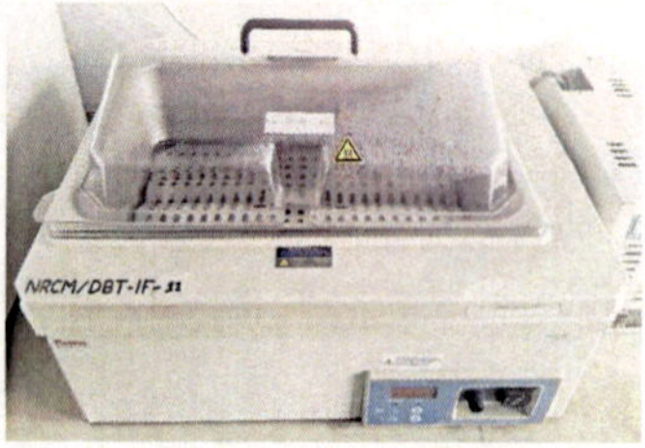

Fig. 26: Water bath

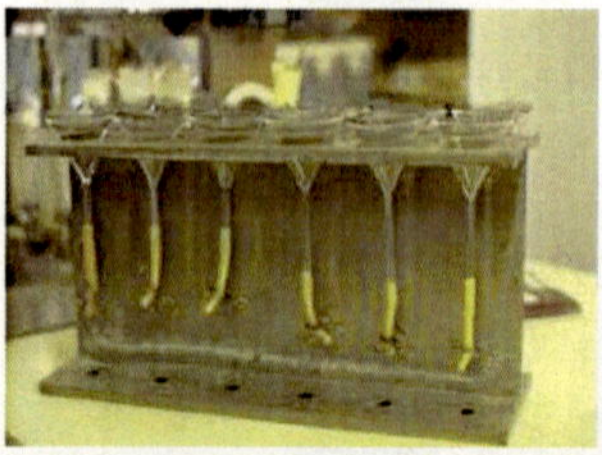

A. Baemann apparatus,

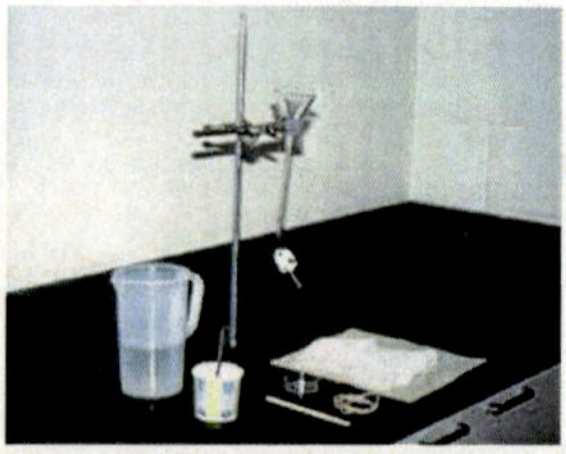

B. Baermann technique and

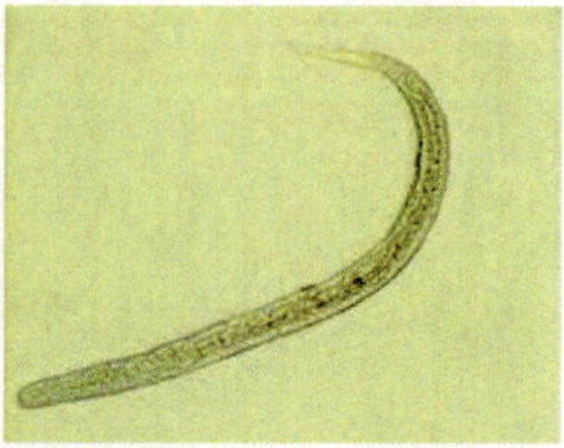

C. Nematode larvae(culture)

Fig. 27

Parasites: at a glance

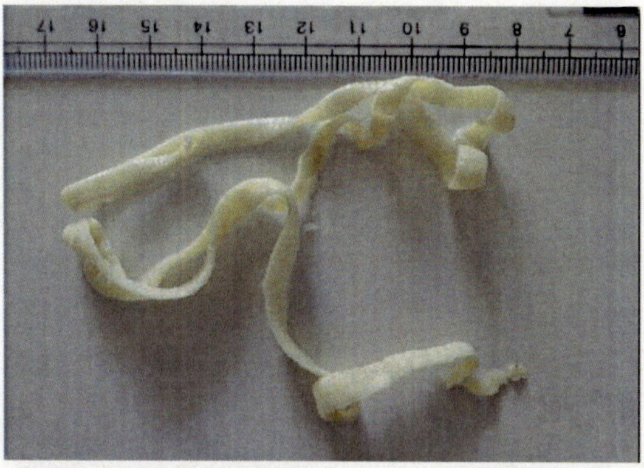

Tape worm (Taenia)

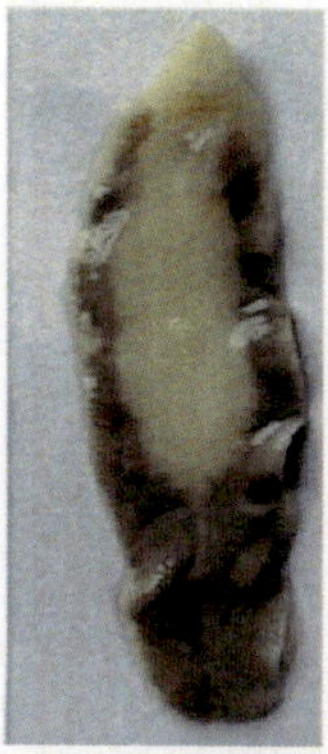

Fluke (Fasciola)

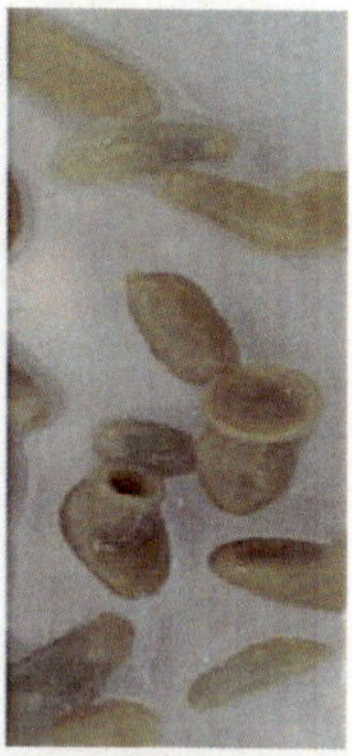

Amphistomes

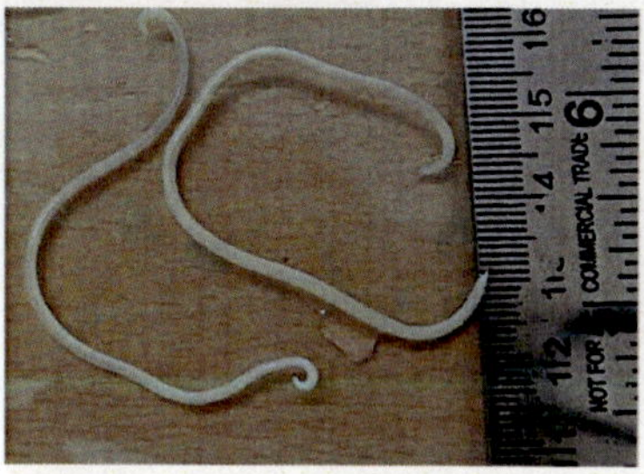

Roundworm (Toxocara)

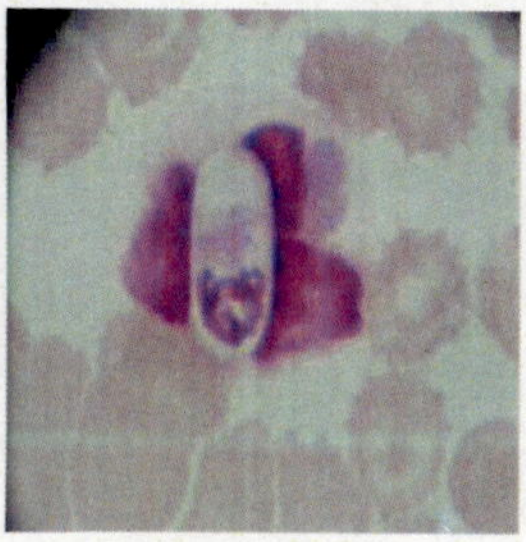

Hepatozoon in neutrophil

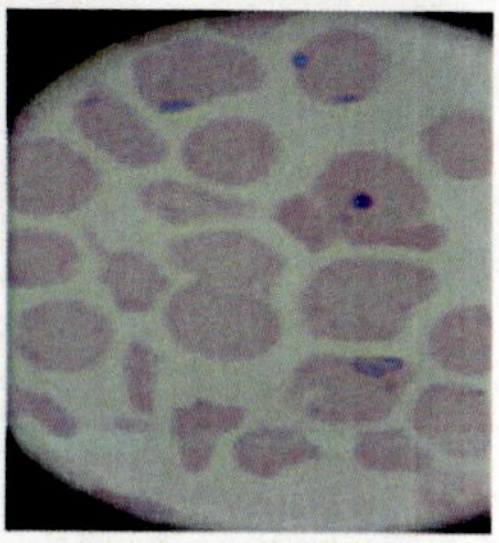

Anaplasma in RBCs

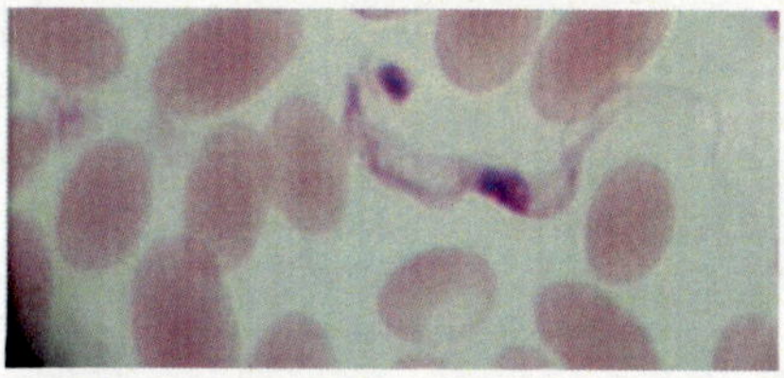

Trypanosoma in blood plasma

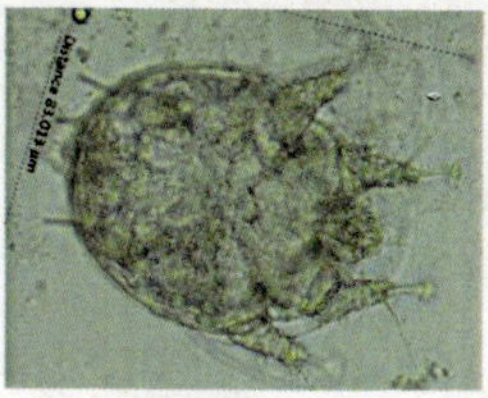

Mites (*Sarcoptes*)

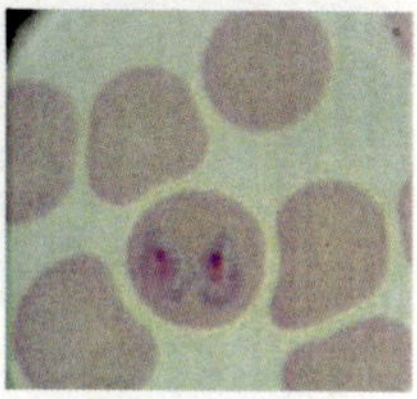

Babesia in RBC

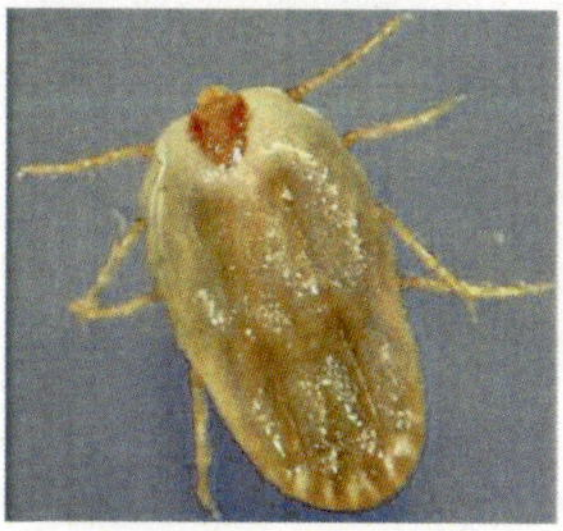

Hard tick (Rhipicephalus microplus) Female

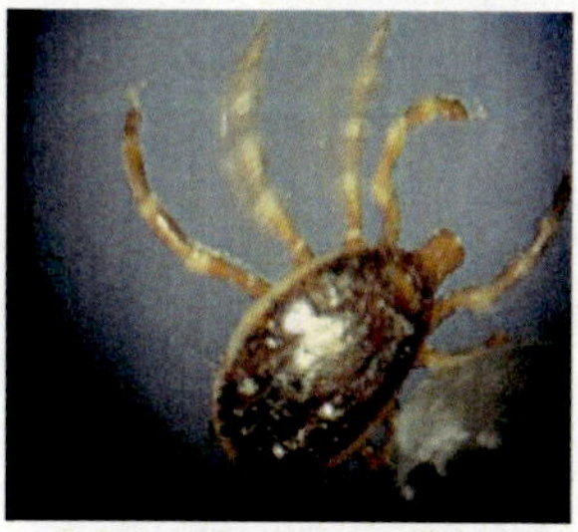

Hard tick (*Hyalomma* spp.) Male

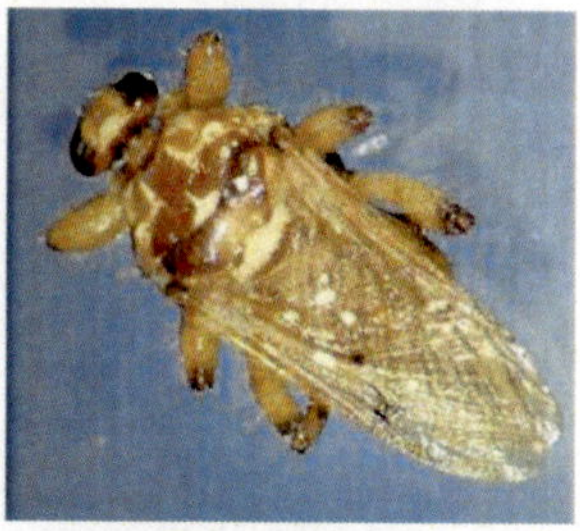

Flies (*Hippobosca*)

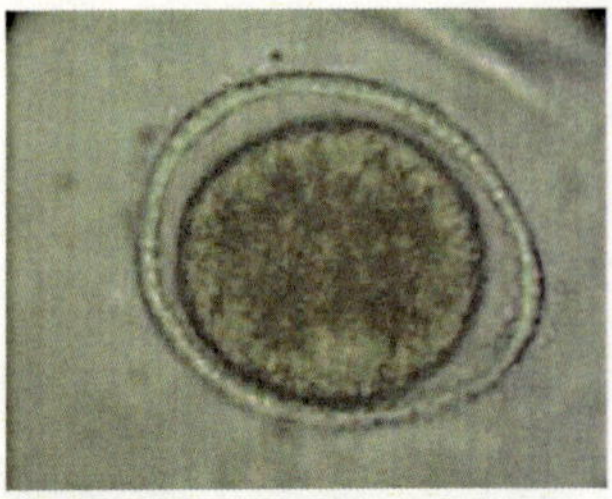
Ascarid eggs (Toxocara)

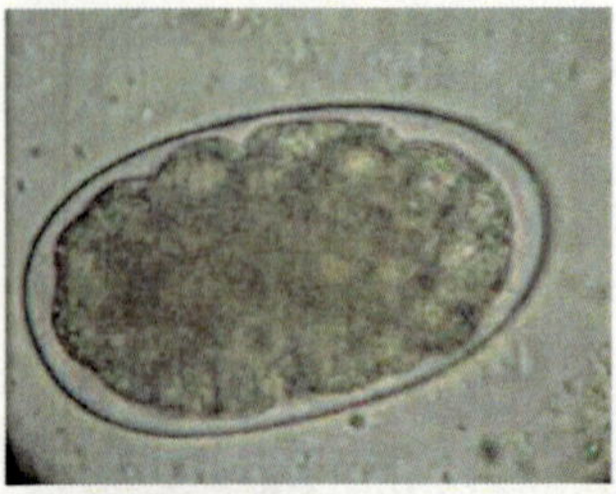
Strongyle eggs

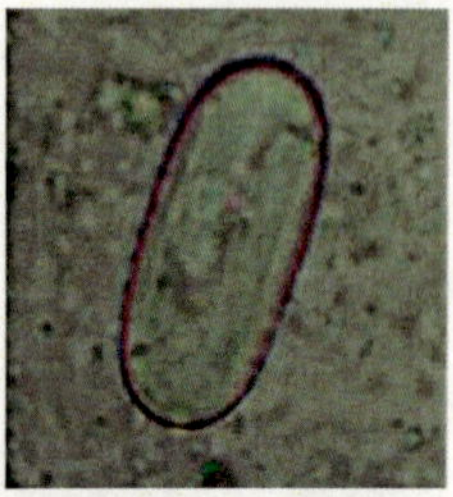
Spirurid egg (*Spirocerca*)

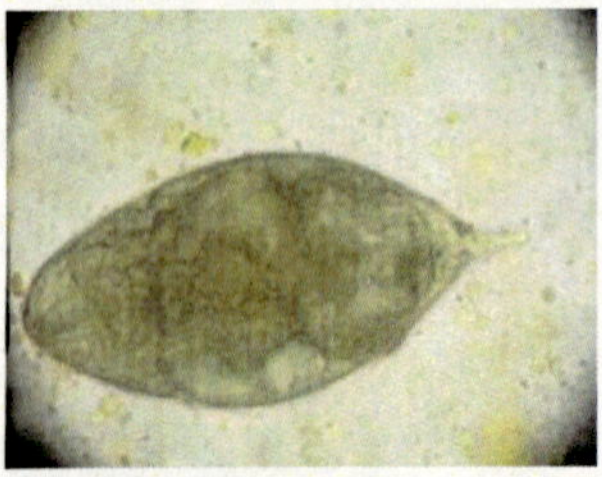
Pseudoparasite

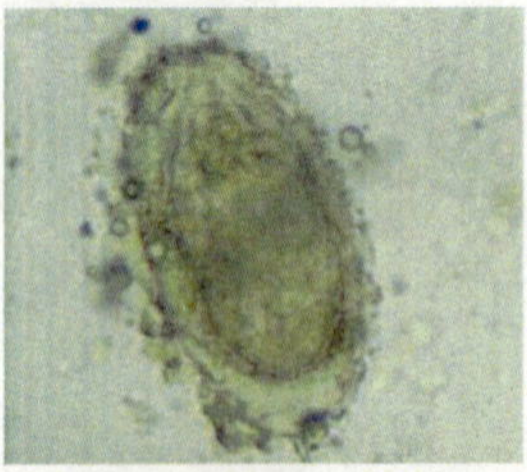
Schis tosoma egg

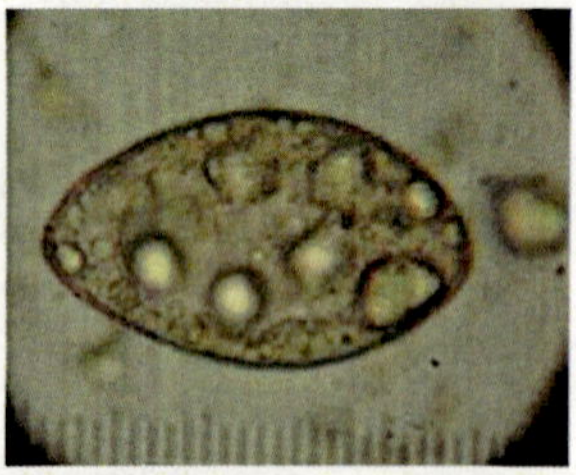
Egg (*Spirometra*)

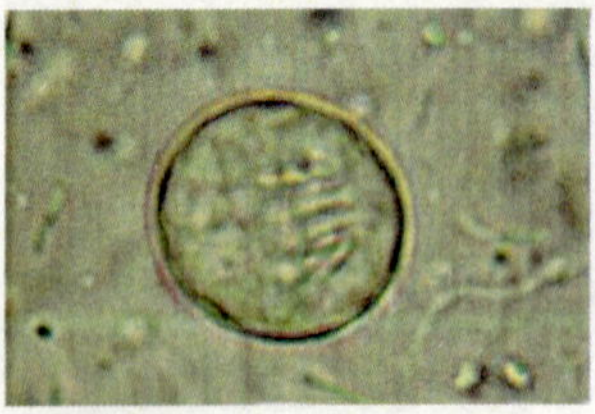
Egg (*Taenia*)

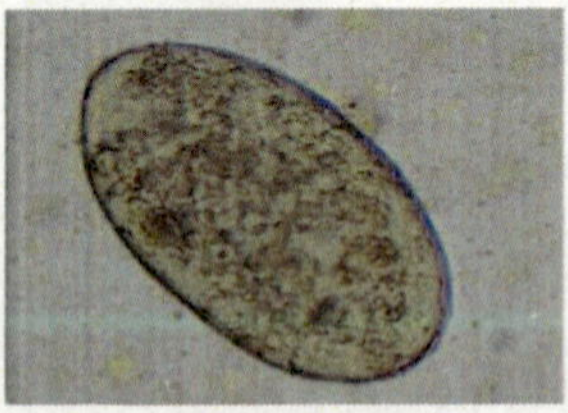
Egg (Amphistome)

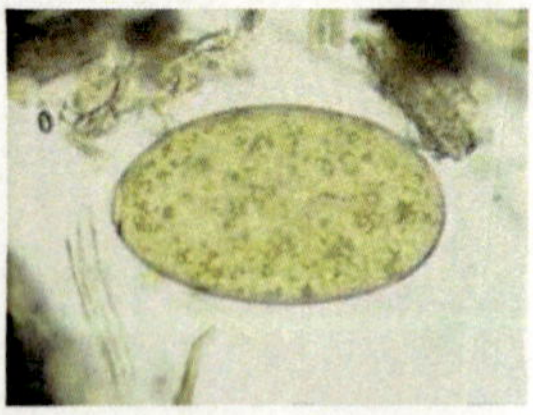
Egg (*Fasciola*)

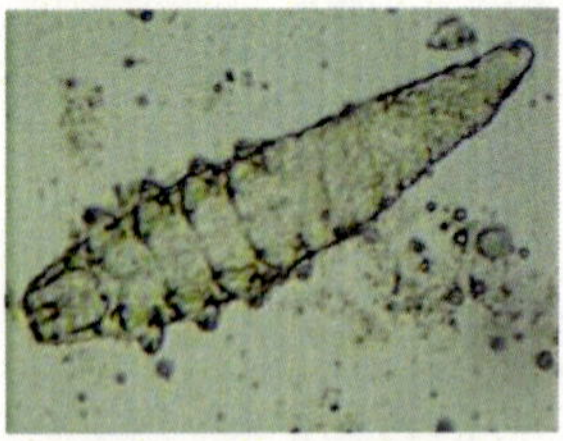
Adult mite (*Demodex*)

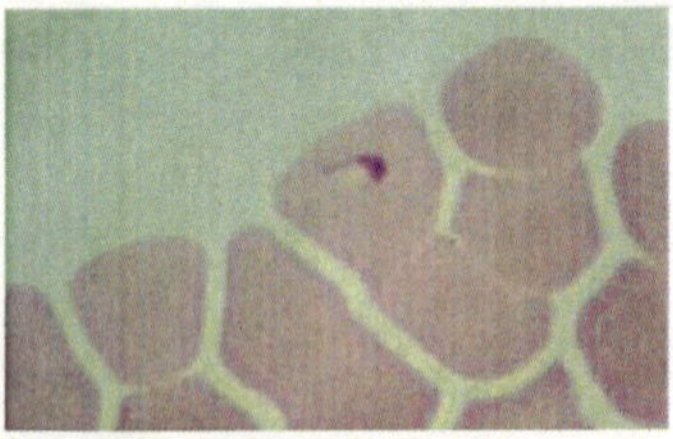
Theileria in RBC

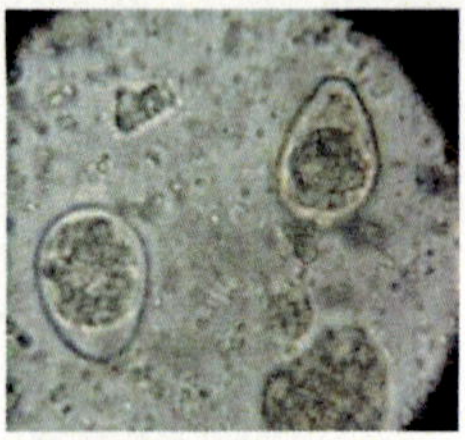
Coccidian oocyst (unsporulated)

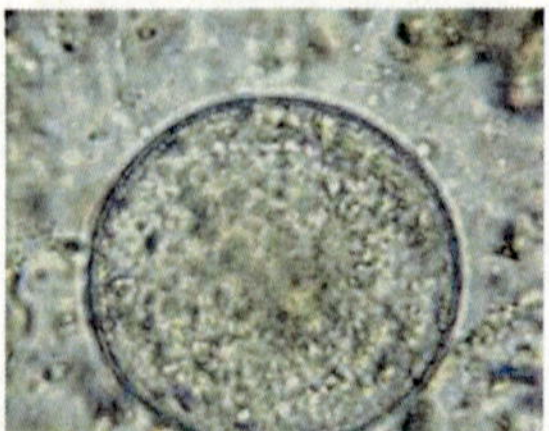
Cyst (*Buxtonella*)

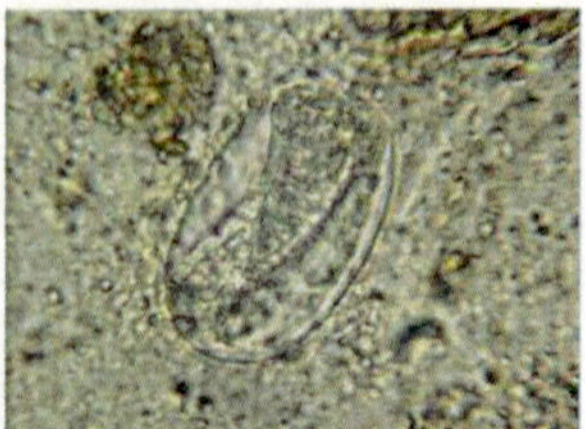
Egg containing Larvae (Strongyloides)

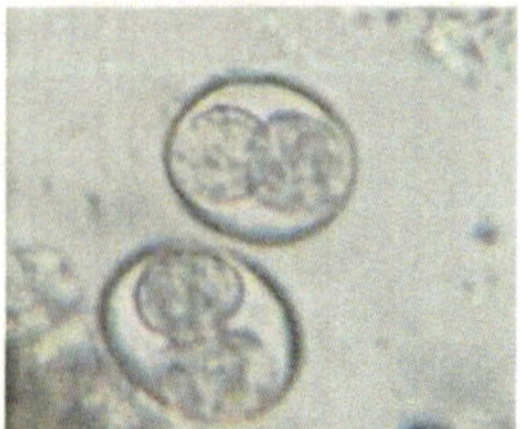
Coccidian oocyst sporulated)

Index